You **can** choose to

BE IN CHARGE

of yourself and your health

IT'S FREE OF CHARGE

by

Dino Georgalas

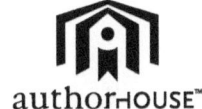

authorHOUSE™

1663 LIBERTY DRIVE, SUITE 200
BLOOMINGTON, INDIANA 47403
(800) 839-8640
WWW.AUTHORHOUSE.COM

First published by AuthorHouse 07/29/05

ISBN: 1-4208-1158-4 (e)
ISBN: 1-4208-1159-2 (sc)

Library of Congress Control Number: 2004099403

Printed in the United States of America
Bloomington, Indiana

This book is printed on acid-free paper.

"KNOW THYSELF"

An inscription at the Oracle of Delphi, as per Plutarch, a second century BC Greek academician and member of the Oracle of Delphi Priesthood College

To remind all the "Big Bang" compadres, young and old,
that we are each one of a kind, and of our inherent and absolute Free Will/Power of Choice, and in particular
those struggling with stress, poor health, obesity, depression, and/or plain life angst and anguish.

To my daughter, Katja, for her insight and appreciation
of our Power of Choice, as well as her devotion to the healing principle of a Healthy Mind in a Healthy Body.

Be in Charge, It's Free of Charge
INTRODUCTION

BE IN CHARGE, IT'S FREE OF CHARGE is about YOU and dedicated to you uniquely. It is but a simple reminder of the uniqueness of each human being and his or her inherent and absolute free will/power of choice. It is based on knowledge/information, be it historical and/or scientific, and observations available to most if not all, as well as basic common sense and logic, not abstractions. It also fully identifies with contemporary and current events with a touch of humor here and there.

This reminder is not an imposition or dogma, be it religious, ideological, spiritual, or other. It does not consist of any instructions or to-do lists of any kind. Nor is it moralizing or judgmental. Nothing is qualified with the words "good," "bad," "right," and "wrong" in this book. It is merely an invitation to *"Know Thyself"* and remember *Thy* inherent and absolute free will/ power of choice that may tangibly empower you to take charge of yourself, your life, and your health, if you so choose.

This power of choice, if one chooses to *Be in Charge* of it, may lead to liberty, a healthy mind in a healthy body, and joy. Simply put, it is a stress-free celebration of a healthy joyful life at *No Charge* and no effort. Just *Being in Charge* of yourself may well do it.

TABLE OF CONTENTS

1 - RIGHT AFTER YOU, THE MOLD WAS BROKEN

Law enforcement and judicial authorities became much more effective once the fingerprint comparison science was introduced, based on the fact that no two fingerprints are alike. DNA and eye scanning comparisons further amplified the effectiveness of our security and our judicial systems. They are based on the fact that no two sets are alike. There will probably be even more such biometric comparison tools used in the future, which will confirm the uniqueness of each individual, particularly with the advent of increased terrorism and computer crime.

Heracleitus, the fifth century BC Greek philosopher, concluded that *everything* in the Universe is perpetually in constant motion. Similar conclusions were made by others who followed Heracleitus, including Einstein and continuing all the way to current science. This constant motion evidently provides constant change. It may be said that the only thing that does not change in the Universe is change itself; it is always ongoing.

As a result of this constant motion and change, Heracleitus stated, *"You cannot step in the same river twice,"* i.e., identical duplication is impossible in the Universe, or as Yogi Berra may have put it, *"You couldn't clone a Xerox copy if your life depended on it."*

Each one of us is therefore UNIQUE just as if, when

we were made or created, the mold was instantly broken. This uniqueness is amplified by our lifestyles, our environment, and our experiences, etc. Could it be that the uniqueness of fingerprints, DNA, etc., is but a confirmation of Heracleitus' musing about stepping into a river?

Any "One-Size-Fits-All" doctrine must, therefore, be an oxymoron and a MYTH at best.

Plain, old, common sense has always had an inkling of this, and over time people came up with popular common sense expressions such as:

- To each his own.

- One man's meat, another man's poison.

- It is in the eyes of the beholder.

- Different strokes for different folks.

- A thousand monks, a thousand religions (old Tibetan monk saying), etc., etc.

Generalizations, of course, are not only an "inexact science," but inherently illogical as well. They do, however, serve to add color and enliven discussions, debates, etc. They are often a summary of personal subjective impressions, and as long as they do not translate into inflexible preconceptions, such as One-Size-Fits-All approaches, they can be somewhat inconsequential.

It would appear that we are, and have been, besieged for quite a while by the determined and all-encompassing myth of One-Size-Fits-All, and anyone opposing it may risk being ostracized, with compliance being promoted as the only salvation, i.e., continuous and total admiration of the Emperor's New Clothes or else.

The apparent, continuous, and holistic carpet bombardment by the myth has affected all facets and aspects of society: what we should eat and drink and when, how to exercise, what to wear, what to drive, what fun is supposed to be, and on and on. And the most tragically pernicious effect seems to have been on our physical and mental health, as well as the quality of our health care and its costs; just look around and behold the devastation.

Not too long ago some advertising media gurus publicly bragged that all they need is thirty seconds on TV to make the public, which might be by now already preconditioned, do anything they want it to do.

Were Pavlov and Goebbels around nowadays, they would probably be experiencing multiple orgasms non-stop, while making more money than the ex-CEOs of Enron, Tyco, etc., without even having to cook the books.

Once upon a time in our free democratic society, which is based on supply and demand capitalism, advertising consisted of just providing simple awareness, i.e., "This is what we are offering, and these are the available options at these prices, and if any of the above turns you on, we will only be too happy to wrap it." A figurative version of the current situation, however, may bring to mind what Schultz and Klink might have uttered in a Hogan's Heroes episode, "You veel do vat vee tell you, venn vee tell you, and you veel like it and you veel enjoy it."

Maybe John Stuart Mill, the nineteenth century British philosopher economist, had a point when he stated, *"Whatever crushes individuality is despotism, by whatever name it may be called."*

Sporadically, some public outcry surfaces (mostly too little and too late) routinely demanding additional government regulation and/or legal action. In time, and at this pace, we may end up even regulating blinking in public within a tort Valhalla environment. Meanwhile, the myth continues to thrive as frustration and despair are amplified. Obviously, this is not the answer to this oxymoron myth, which WE allow to aggress us and invade us.

The answer lies uniquely within each one of us, individually, and absolutely nowhere else. Just like faith, it lies in our heart and mind, not inside a cathedral, mosque, synagogue, temple, or elsewhere. Nor is it dependent on something or somebody else and their actions.

Undoubtedly, we will eventually get back in the saddle and that may be sooner rather than later, as Americans by and large seem to be generously endowed with common sense and practicality. All there is to it is for each one of us to remember our UNIQUENESS.

Since one size does not fit all, generalizations may

tend to also be oxymorons. That is why it is being deliberately and repeatedly stated here that: "one may or could," or "you or we may or could," or "some may or could." It is merely to emphasize that, "*If* the shoe (of *your* choice) fits, then you may try wearing it if *you* so *choose*." These seemingly ambiguous repetitions are not intended to come across as "Shakespearean" or "Dickensian" nuances, but merely as constant reminders that the ONE SIZE **DOES NOT** FIT ALL (as each one of us is unique) and that the choice is strictly and individually yours/ours at all times and never anybody else's.

2 - BAAANG!!! ... AND HERE WE ARE

It has been a while since scientists came up with the Big Bang thesis, which is the somehow "accidental" explosion that produced the Universe, and all the equally accidental consequences going all the way to Darwin and beyond.

Genesis aside, questions, speculations, and controversy hounded the experts for a long, long time regarding how, who, or what created the Universe, and whether the Big Bang explosion was an accident, or whether it was caused by an extra-cosmic McVeigh or Bin Laden. Some even toyed with the God idea.

More recently, scientists benefiting from our most advanced space exploration, i.e., satellites, space stations, Hubble telescopes, etc., seem to have reached a new conclusion, as reported by various media and which may be so summarized. The Big Bang does not seem to be accidental anymore. It seems that the resulting precise GRAVITY and the ever-evolving after effects of this unimaginably designed explosion or Big Bang were predetermined with absolute precision, balance, and control, down to the minutest subatomic particle as well as its pre-programmed, perpetually organized constant motion, evolution, and expansion. So much for Darwin's "micro-organisms" that had unprotected sex on their honeymoon in the Galapagos way back when.

Scientists, therefore, concluded that only some inconceivable intelligence could be the culprit that organized the whole thing, but they have no clue as to the identity of that intelligence. Some folks, including some scientists, jumped on the God Idea Bandwagon. That, of course, is a no-no for some fans of the Ninth Circuit Court of Appeals in California, which while contemplating our pledge of allegiance, declared God unconstitutional, since *"God could be easily substituted for Zeus."*

That, however, would be comparing apples and oranges. For one thing, two millennia ago God purportedly had an only child, who was born in the "West Bank," while Zeus, an inveterate cosmic Casanova, had gazillions of kids all over the cosmos for much longer than 2000 years, not to mention that his Mount Olympus budget is permanently in the red due to his child support program overruns.

In his desperate efforts to balance his budget, Zeus could get some temporary relief by contracting with Arthur Andersen's consulting as well as their auditing services, while supplementing his revenues with Viagra endorsements. One would think that with his prestige and "potent" reputation he could easily "outgun" Bob Dole and even Slick Willy (Bob's partner in *60 Minutes*) as the Viagra poster boy. Not that he personally needs the pills. Interestingly enough, following the inaugural appearance of Bob & Bill on *60 Minutes*, Jay Leno commented, *"One is on Viagra, the other IS Viagra."* Apparently, neither Zeus nor anybody in the audience had any questions about "What IS, IS."

8

In deference, however, to some of the Ninth Circuit Court fans, who may be known as Zeus Club members, we could temporarily at least, name the intelligence responsible for the Big Bang that the scientists could not identify. "UBB" is short for Unidentified Big Banger, while for some God might be more acceptable, and for yet some others OUI, which is short for Organization Universe Inc., may be more appropriate, and they could all be interchangeable in order to satisfy as many as possible. But, please, no Zeus.

One look at humans, our world, and our Universe, and one may find these creations quite awesome and beyond imagination or expression, except for saying, "GREAT JOB UBB, WELL DONE."

Some could, if somewhat selfishly if not, arrogantly consider humans as the most magnificent creation in the universe. Sophocles, the celebrated fifth century BC Greek poet and dramatist, agreed, as he stated, *"Wonders are many, and none is more wonderful than man."* For the benefit of the Ninth Circuit Court fans, we could call this UBB's most magnificent creation, a bio-chemical, electro-mechanical contraption that is a self-sustaining, self-regenerating, self-repairing, self-healing and self-computing "Gizmo of Ultimate Perfection," or GUP for short. And let's pray that neither Microsoft nor IBM file with the Ninth Circuit for any unconstitutional patent infringements.

From time immemorial, and through countless civilizations, human beings have been aware that they inherently, have a free will. Even in the Garden of Eden, nobody and nothing tried to stop Eve from serving a Martha Stewart apple pie to her boyfriend. Our founding fathers also, ensconced our inherent free will in the declaration of independence and our Constitution, and as they said, "*It is self-evident…,*"

If you think about it, you may very well conclude, "Only **YOU** can think the thoughts **YOU** (choose to) think, Only **YOU** can speak the words **YOU** (choose to) speak, Only **YOU** can do the deeds **YOU** (choose to) do, and **NEVER** <u>anybody else</u>!."

How is that for self-evident?

Let us recap the self-evident "specs" of UBB's most wondrous creation, human beings, a.k.a. GUPs, which are possibly "created in his or her image and/or as his or her personal expression."

1 Each one of us is unique.

2 Each one of us has been blessed with the gift of discrimination.

3 Each one of us is endowed with the Free Will/ Power of Choice.

4 We are all created equal.

5 We all have access to equal opportunity.

(Maybe the EEOC could put in a favourable word to the Ninth Circuit Court, i.e., that God a.k.a. UBB, is OK as an equal opportunity supporter as opposed to Zeus).

In case anybody wonders why God/UBB "did not go

all the way," and provide equal outcome as well, the clear answer is that he would have had to cancel out our Free Will/Power of Choice, but evidently chose not to. However, there was someone much later who promised a guaranteed equal outcome to all, "Slick Vlad," a.k.a. Lenin and consequently he did everything he could to wipe out free will everywhere he could for about seventy-five years, and without ever delivering the goodies.

The cosmologists who came up with UBB had focused on the law of Gravity of the Universe, and before them Einstein concentrated on the law of Relativity as well as the Unified Field. Another very important and self-evident law of the Universe is the law of Cause and Effect, i.e., as everything in the underlying energy "grid" of the Universe (no more visible to the human eye than gravity), is "interwoven," and nothing can take place anywhere without affecting something else, somehow, somewhere, in the Universe. Since fundamentally everything is energy, it means that our every thought, word, and deed, **always** affects something else, somehow, somewhere, i.e., there are always "inevitable/natural" consequences. Therefore, through our Free Will/Power of Choice, we can always choose our thoughts, words, and deeds, and, therefore, also their "inevitable/natural" consequences as well. Simply put, We can Be In Charge of Ourselves, if we Choose to.

Being mindful of the law of Cause and Effect, when we exercise our Free Will/Power of Choice , it means that we choose to have, as well, a "say" in the consequences of our thoughts, words, and deeds. This "say" may be commonly described as responsibility.

When you are responsible, then you are the Boss of Yourself. On the other hand if, when we exercise our Free Will/Power of Choice we do not take into consideration the law of Cause and Effect, it simply means that we choose not to have a "say" in the consequences, which is commonly described as irresponsibility. When you are irresponsible, you simply are not the Boss of Yourself. Being responsible means we are in charge of the consequences, and not the other way around. We can, therefore, be our own Boss all the time when we so Choose.

The amount of LIBERTY provided by our Free Will/ Power of Choice is commensurate to how mindful we are of the law of Cause and Effect, i.e., the amount of responsibility we choose to exercise. The more we are responsible then the freer we are. Responsibility is to liberty what breathing is to our lungs.

Liberty has been forever cherished by humanity, and amply available to the responsible. Our founding fathers, who appreciated liberty, expressed it magnificently through their spokesman Patrick Henry who said, *"Give Me Liberty Or Give Me Death.."*

3 -CHOICES "À LA CARTE"

Since the Universe and everything in it is in constant motion and change, then it inherently provides us non-stop new/different "situations," i.e., fresh choices every instant. Our inherent Free Will/Power of Choice is never, never switched off; it seems inextricably and permanently "hardwired" in us. No amount of rationalization and/or denial will "unplug" it. Throughout our lives we keep making Choices non-stop, whether we acknowledge them or not, or whether we attribute them to somebody else or not, or whether we deny them or not. Denying our Free Will/Power of Choice is merely an act of self-deception, which is also our choice.

Some of the most common verbalizations of our Free Will/Power of Choice and attempts at denial seem to be the following:

1   *"I had no choice."* This canonized oxymoron is always eloquently accompanied by a myriad of futile rationalizations to justify self-fooling.

2   *"It is God's Will."* This is a passing of the buck again, to the Guy or Gal Upstairs. But maybe His or Her will is our will since He/She gave us Free Will/Power of Choice in the first place compliments of the Big Bang, It doesn't get any plainer than this.

3   *"It is not my fault."* In the old blame game everything is always everybody and everything else's fault.

4 *"The devil made me do it."* This ageless classic stand-by is promoted by Adam and Eve in the "Original Sin" infomercial starring the snake.

Any of the above thoughts, and their resulting words and deeds, as well as the consequences thereof, are always chosen by none other than you, and denying this self-evident fact is self-deception and a denial of responsibility and, therefore, a deterioration of your liberty, not to mention an over abundance of self-induced and perniciously hazardous stress. Should you not choose death over the loss of your liberty, not to worry. The stress you choose instead, may eventually do you in anyway, and more painfully at that, not to mention suffering, agony, and the "privilege" of exorbitant healthcare bills.

Denying our Free Will/Power of Choice may not be unlike racing an Indy 500 car and tossing out the steering wheel. It is hard to imagine anyone consciously enjoying the agony preceding the crash. You may very well want to hold on to your steering wheel and Be In Charge and enjoy a safe and thrilling ride no matter what, since you are the only one that has a say in this anyway. Vernon Howard expressed it aptly in one of his books, *"Nothing in the Universe can harm you unless you allow it."*

According to Billy, a.k.a. the Bard, *"The whole world is a stage and every man and woman merely players, etc."* But, once the Free Will/Power of Choice is factored in, then the players may very well, also, become simultaneously directors and producers. If Billy was still with us today, and a Trekkie at that, he would maybe change his statement to, "The whole world is a "Holodeck," like the one on Captain Jean Luc Picard's *Enterprise*.

From the moment we emerge from the womb, we are constantly flooded with other people's information, opinions, dogmas, habits, etc., and as we grow, we acquire our own knowledge and accumulate experience. As we evolve however, at times it's still quite a challenge to distinguish between our very own thoughts and experiences, and those of others which we may have adopted and may have automatically claimed as our very own. Such confusing data, and at times contradictory data, may undermine our goals and/or direction when we exercise our Free Will/ Power of Choice, and may very well create internal conflict. Some may have eventually discovered, through experience, that such "foreign" confusing data had been very limiting and conveyed an impression of being chain bound by self imposed limitations.

When exercising our Free Will/Power of Choice, in order to focus on our own knowledge, experience, thoughts, and beliefs, and not someone else's, we may vet them first to ensure genuine ownership or as Ronnie put it to Mikhail, *"We Trust But Verify."* Finally, you may want to double check by getting a stamp of approval of your feelings/instincts, which is sort of like the seal of Good Housekeeping. The farmers are right on, as they keep insisting on separating the wheat from the chaff. Some may find it quite helpful to always remember that there is NO such a thing as "good" and "bad" choices. There are only the choices that people make, and which they acknowledge they made, and the choices they make and deny they made.

<u>But they did make them all!</u>

The following ten tips, hints, and reminders, may prove helpful to some in exercising their Free Will/Power of Choice to its fullest potential, easily and assuredly should they choose to:

1   Remember *who you are*.

2   Observe like Sherlock Holmes, or as Yogi Berra put it, *"You can sometimes see a lot just by looking,"* and had Sherlock overheard him then he might have muttered to his acolyte, *"Elementary, my dear Watson."*

3   Seek out what is really what. Just as Jack Webb, Dragnet's original Joe Friday put it, *"Just the facts, mam."*

4   Run them down and check them out as doggedly as Detective Columbo.

5   Reduce them down to the lowest common denominator. That World War I British general hit the nail on the head when he said on a French battlefield, *"Keep It Simple Stupid."* Today we recognize it as the "KISS" principle.

6   Base your choice on what would benefit *Numero Uno* the most (that means **YOU**), to empower **YOU** to "Be All **YOU** Can Be." It looks like the Marine Corps recruiters are in agreement and always "Semper Fi." In Captain Kirk terminology, this could read as *"The Prime Directive."*

7 **Will it provide you with joy**? If affirmative, proceed.

8 ***Will it benefit others as well?*** If affirmative, proceed.

9 Enlist the support and confirmation of your feelings/ instincts.

10 Lastly, pedal to the metal, **CHOOSE.** Then charge head on with passion and joy, as you cannot miss unless you choose to.

Who you are.

- We are all part of this Universe. (Big Bang or no Big Bang).

- Each one of us is unique.

- Each one of us has the gift of discrimination.

- Each one of us is endowed with the absolute inherent Free Will/Power of Choice

- We are all created Equal.

- We all have equal opportunity.

Numero Uno.

Numero Uno is your top priority, never mind the routine mantra "others come first," or "self-sacrifice for the benefit of others," etc. You cannot boost a stranded motorist's battery unless yours is in ship shape in the first place, or else you will both be stranded.

Will Others Benefit As Well?

We are all inextricably intertwined; the underlying energy of the Universe took care of that. Furthermore, by looking around, an observer may well realize that a deal is not a deal unless it is "WIN, WIN" for all concerned. Not everybody has to win equally, and so long as there is no loser it is a win. Only Lenin promised that all would win equally. Promises, promises.

4 - CHOOSING TO SABOTAGE YOUR OWN FREE WILL/POWER OF CHOICE

Denial of one's inherent, absolute Free Will/Power of Choice, invariably leads to the ultimate and insidious self-deception, i.e., denying that the Free Will/Power of Choice is ours and ours alone. Denial of responsibility is the natural and inevitable consequence of this self-deception.

DENIAL OF RESPONSIBILITY seems to be the most fundamental expression of our choosing not to recognize and acknowledge our inherent Free Will/Power of Choice. Its *rewards* are suppression of liberty and lots and lots of stress.

Since at the core of our denial of responsibility is the denial of our Free Will/Power of Choice, it means it is also the denial of the consequences of our choices, which is irresponsibility, and it comes in various insidious shapes and forms.

As honest Abe said:

- ***"You can fool some of the people all the time, you can fool all the people some of the time, but you cannot fool all the people all the time."***

Also, epitomizing what Lincoln said:

- *"And at no time can you fool yourself; all attempts to do so may prove painful and hazardous to your health."*

Choosing to fool one's self is the most insidious form of irresponsibility. It includes lying to yourself as well as others. Lying is an attempt to deny the existence of truth, and that is one big exercise in futility. Truth is here, there, and everywhere, coexisting with everything else in the Universe, and goes on and on, and just as eternal. It just hangs out there, and to some it might look like the sword of Damocles, as illustrated by the "Enron Tapes" that surfaced years after the scandal broke. Some may conclude that if you keep on and on, rationalizing something, it is probably a lie in the first place.

Lying can be very, very frustrating because it is extremely hard work, around the clock 24/7, and requires extraordinary memory. Furthermore, it is futile and its wages are stress and fear, in particular, the constant fear of being found out. All that effort and stress for nothing; the truth will always be there anyway. That does not necessarily mean that only the scared and lazy folks with memory lapses are truthful. It simply means that those who love liberty, rather than stress, may always choose truth. The Great Iconoclast from Nazareth was most certainly not kidding when he said, *"AND THE TRUTH SHALL SET YOU FREE."* He sure knew his stuff.

According to Elbert Hubbard, *"FREEDOM IS THE SUPREME GOOD... FREEDOM FROM SELF IMPOSED LIMITATION."*

Lying may be the mother of all self-imposed limitations.

Accordingly, lying or fooling yourself is oxymoronic and therefore destroys your freedom and creates stressful self-contradiction and the resulting internal conflict, which is the primary source of human stress. It is extremely toxic and hazardous to your mental and physical health. Stress, following insufferable pain, can ultimately kill, and it does kill as continuously reconfirmed by the latest medical findings.

An appropriate figurative illustration can be found in some of the original Star Trek episodes. Particularly, the episode where captain Kirk is faced with "Nomad" an all powerful and invincible robotic entity that has gone haywire, and is now bent on destroying the "Enterprise," Earth, and other planetary systems sustaining "imperfect" human life. Helpless, Captain Kirk could not neutralize "Nomad." In desperation, he managed to get it to contradict itself, and be in conflict with its mission. It soon started to mumble, stutter, smoke, hiss, spark, and fizzle out, all the way to self-destruction. Similar parallel scenarios appeared in other Kirk episodes. The non-Trekkies on the other hand, may instead visualize Michael Schumacher trying to win a F-1 Grand Prix race, while flooring simultaneously the gas and brake pedals, as team Ferrari contemplates hara-kiri.

Although we do not spark and hiss like "Nomad" or blow pistons like a race car, we also may self-destruct from within. Medical science keeps on reconfirming the devastation human stress inflicts on our physical and mental health. Obviously, the avoidance of contradicting ourselves, and the resulting inner conflicts may do wonders for our health, quality of life, and our pocket books, at the very least. Tragically, some, and not just the masochists, may believe that stress is unavoidable and beyond their control.

Harry, the spunky fellow from the *"Show Me"* state, expressed it beautifully: *"THE BUCK STOPS HERE!!!"* He proved it time and again during his presidency. It applies to all of us, not just Presidents from Missouri, if we choose to embrace it. Just picture how liberating and empowering it may be, not to mention stress free.

It has often been said that our Creator (take your pick: God, UBB, or Organization Universe Inc.) is the Alpha and the Omega of all creation. We may have very well been empowered by our own free will to be our very own Alpha and Omega, or as Yogi Berra may have put it, "YOU ARE IT."

Philosophers, through the ages, proclaimed that man's greatest challenge is mastery of himself. ***"HE WHO MASTERS HIMSELF, MASTERS THE UNIVERSE."*** Did not the Great Master from Nazareth say something to this effect: *WHAT I DO YOU CAN DO ALSO.* Some may feel that what was left unsaid was *In time, when you will manage to take charge and master yourselves.*

The primal and ultimate irresponsibility is the denial of the Free Will/Power of Choice and the Law Of Cause And Effect. It may very well be easier to quit breathing. Apt illustrations of irresponsibility are the recent seisms that shook our business world, our country, and even the globe, i.e. Enron, Worldcom, Tyco, and Arthur Andersen, just to name a few business giants as well as various Wall Street financial institutions. The resulting "tidal wave" was but a gigantic LOSE, LOSE, (it definitely was not WIN, WIN) exercise. Nobody was spared including the very CEOs, CFOs, etc., that *allegedly* swindled billions.

It would seem that one of the main, if not the main, goal of this particular "Tsunami" of irresponsibility was the excessive and out of control amassing of possessions, while ignoring the obvious; that wealth is measured by "needs" not possessions.

During the fourth century BC, Alexander the Great, the wealthiest and most powerful man of his era, had been impressed by the reputation of the famous cynic philosopher Diogenes, and decided to pay him a visit. On a bright sunny Mediterranean morning, Alexander stood in front of Diogenes, who was sitting outside his "mansion" (an oversized clay jar) enjoying the sun, and said to him, *"Diogenes, I am Alexander the Great. Name anything you would like and it shall be yours."* And Diogenes responded, *"Step aside, you are blocking the sun."* It would seem that Diogenes was the wealthiest of the two, not to mention the fact that he would not have been a VIP client of the IRS either. If one's "needs" exceed one's possessions, there will always be a pool of red ink, which is common sense Accounting 101. Billy the Bard makes the point as well in Richard III, when the king cries, *"My kingdom for a horse."*

More recently, during the Wall Street Seisms, the media reported that a CEO allegedly, in addition to bilking shareholders and employees of hundreds of millions, had been compensating himself with more hundreds of millions, and felt the need to break the law in order to avoid a million and a half in sales taxes. Yet possibly at the same time, a homeless person sleeping overnight on a bench, in a nearby public park, may not have felt so desperately needy as to break the law by cheating and stealing.

Some, of course, blame greed as the culprit, and, therefore, solely responsible, as per the good old "not-my-fault" syndrome. However, Alexander Dumas, you know, the guy who came up with *"Cherchez la femme,"* after having ridden his life's roller coaster for a while, came up with the following, *"Money can be a great servant or a horrible master."* Maybe the prime directive of this horrible master is Greed, but the choice, nevertheless, belongs always, always to each individual.

Just over a year after the Enron scandal broke out, a national daily publication headlined its findings (on a section front page) as follows: "Debt Problems Hit Even The Wealthy," followed by the subheading, "Biggest Surge In Borrowing Is among Those With Highest Incomes." Could this be some sort of reaffirmation that Diogenes is still the wealthiest of the lot, with the least stress, and most liberty?

Socrates, considered by many as the dean of ancient

Greek philosophers, was also a great iconoclast, at least in the minds of the Athenian establishment. Naturally, he was accused and condemned for corrupting the minds of the youth. They, therefore, extended him an invitation he could not refuse to the Areopagus "bar" for cocktails, namely, of the hemlock variety. Maybe at the Areopagos, Athens's Supreme Court, they just did not have at their disposal adequate syringe hygiene, or any appropriately wired chairs or cyanide pellets.

In Socrates' apology, Plato recounts something along these lines. On the eve of Socrates' execution, one of his favourite students and a scion of one of the richest Greek families in Asia Minor, showed up in his prison cell in Athens. After embracing each other with great emotion, the disciple urged Socrates to pack his belongings, as his family's yacht was waiting in Piraeus, and informed him that he had bribed everybody from the coast guard to the prison guard. Once in Asia Minor, he could freely resume teaching philosophy to his heart's content enriching more minds, while living in comfort and security.

Socrates thanked his disciple for the generous offer but declined it, and told him that he would face his executioner in the morning. His disciple was perplexed, and told him that he could not understand his decision, particularly because he had been convicted by a kangaroo court.(Maybe he did not say that exactly, seeing as it was before Captain Cook's cruise down under) on trumped up charges. Socrates responded, that above everything he taught his students, he emphasized the importance to love, honour, and obey, their country at all times. If he would, therefore, escape now, he would be reneging that teaching, thus destroying his own credibility and that of everything he taught, heretofore, and all his efforts would have been for nought, and the injustice of his conviction and condemnation was therefore irrelevant. Next morning, it was all over.

One can appreciate that consequently, and particularly after 33 AD, life insurance premiums for iconoclasts skyrocketed.

Had Yogi Berra been asked to comment on Socrates' last stand, he might have responded,

"HE WALKED THE TALK TILL IT WAS OVER."

Walking the talk is one tangible sign that you are not fooling yourself, or anybody else for that matter, as well as an expression of responsibility. As per the cliche, a picture is worth a thousand words.

But there are never enough words worth a deed.

Deeds are indeed the most powerful teaching tool. Apes seem appreciative as well, hence, "monkey see, monkey do."

As already mentioned, from the second we are born, we are bombarded with all kinds of information and directives with the one underlying command, "That is the way it is or has always been done." It is, therefore, plain but vital common sense, for young children, teenagers, and young adults, to consistently witness parents, educators, community, and business leaders,

WALKING THE TALK. It is the greatest vaccine against self-deception, self-contradiction, internal conflict, and the resulting stress. In other words, there is no room for the timeless classic, "Do as I tell you, not as I do," etc. It could very well ensure that the biblical message, *"the sins of the fathers visit the sons,"* does not materialize accompanied by the resulting internal conflicts and stress.

Also, according to Goethe, *"The Deed Is Everything. Its Repute Nothing."* If one thinks about it, whether on a personal basis or in a leadership role, some may discover that nothing may be more liberating and effective than "*declaring the goal and walking the talk*."

Remember that choosing not to choose is a choice just the same, and as such, a choice that undermines our Free Will/Power of Choice. Denying responsibility is also a choice. According to Billy the Bard, *"To be or not to be, that is the question,"* and a self-evident answer is not both, at least not at the same time. Roy Rogers would have probably confirmed that you cannot simultaneously ride two horses going in different directions. You do not have to be an OBGYN to know that you cannot be pregnant just a little bit, you are either pregnant or not...

"You cannot serve two masters," confirmed the Nazarene Master.

The delusion of choosing not to choose is, to say the least quite, uncomfortable. As ranchers tell it, *"He who sits on the fence too long, gets a sore crotch."*

The Six Most "Popular" Forms of Irresponsibility

Irresponsibility, as some may have noticed, comes in various shapes and forms that one may "choose" from. The following appear to be the six most basic, common, and even popular, derivatives of the denial of one's Free Will/Power of and its natural consequences.

"It's Not My Fault" may be the most elementary form of irresponsibility, and practically a knee jerk reaction for some that may have reached epidemic proportions. "It's not our fault" (*it never is*); it is everybody else's fault; or it is because of this or that. It is as if everybody was automatically and absolutely covered by an imaginary no fault, or rather, a "no responsibility" insurance policy, or infected by a potent "NOT-MY-FAULT" virus.

There is an old saying that reflects on "not-my-fault" attitudes. "When the immature (not to mention morons) are faced with what they view as adverse events, whether of their doing or not, they may blame everybody and everything under the sun except themselves. The semi-mature facing similar adverse events may solely blame themselves. The mature and wise may blame nobody and nothing, but may observe, take notice, and move on." It looks like Vince Lombardi was a member in good standing, of the latter group, since his credo was *"Blame Nothing, Expect Nothing, Do Something."* Both the immature and the wise may make "mistakes." The difference may be that the wise learn from their mistakes.

Pursuit of Excess has been close to the top of the

irresponsibility hit parade for quite a while now. It has been practically institutionalized, maybe even sanctified, with the psalms of MORE IS BETTER, BIGGER IS BETTER, NEWER AND NEWER, MORE AND MORE IMPROVED, etc., etc.

Plato's most famous student, and the mentor of Alexander the Great, was none other than Aristotle, the celebrated fourth century BC philosopher, scientist, and metaphysician. Many may be familiar with the pillar of his teachings, i.e., *"Moderation in everything."* It would seem, though, that for some, moderation is at times associated with wishy-washy, non-committal sitting on the fence, indecisive, wimpy, etc. Aristotle expressed his moderation philosophy quite laconically in just three words. An attempt at a literal translation, also in three words comes up with, *"ALL MEASURE EXCELS,"* Measure meaning the achievement of a "golden" balance, or equilibrium between excesses and that which is always OPTIMAL. Remember the folks who could not identify UBB, how amazed they were by the perfectly BALANCED results of the Big Bang, i.e., our UNIVERSE.

Many may agree, therefore, that there is nothing wishy-washy, indecisive, or wimpy, about an airline pilot keeping the plane level (balanced) in flight. On the other hand, excesses are not unlike cruising down the turnpike at the wheel of an eighteen-wheeler and jerking the steering wheel lock to lock non-stop. The agonizing outcome is best left to one's imagination. It might at times rhyme with Newton's law, which says, *"To every action there is an equal and opposite* *reaction." Maybe the Founding Fathers did appreciate Aristotle's point of view and enriched the Constitution with Checks and **Balances.***

Excesses, like everything else, are also governed by the law of Cause and Effect. Excesses and their consequences may be quite visible to anyone that chooses to observe. They are all around us, affecting our lifestyles, our health, our environment, our occupations, etc., provided we choose to allow them to affect us.

The oxymoron aspect of excess may be illustrated by this anecdote on the ever increasing multiplication of specialists. Specialization has been defined, by some, as the art or science of knowing more and more about less and less. It may very well be that The ultimate (excessive) specialist "knows everything about nothing." Excess begats excess.

The recent well-publicized disastrous scandals in the corporate, financial, and stock market worlds, that rocked the country are also the results of excess, e.g., who will merge or acquire the most, whose stock will climb the most and fastest, who will have the most sales, who will post the most profits (real or unreal), etc., etc., including, or rather concluding in, who will commit more and bigger fraud. Some may call this being competitive, so were the kamikaze pilots until they ended up losers. It may seem at times that excess has become a goal in itself. A glance at the post-Enron national socio-economic environment may indicate that Aristotle had a point after all.

Diogenes, the same guy who told Alexander the Great where to go, once wondered at high noon in mid-summer with a lit lantern in the market place of ancient Athens. Eventually, he was asked what the heck he thought he was doing, and he replied, *"I am looking for an honest man."* Just imagine if nowadays, Diogenes and his lantern (make it a solar powered flashlight) would pull the same stunt in Wall Street in the wake of all business excesses authored by the various "Saddams" of the corporate, financial, and investment worlds. He would probably collapse, with frustration and exhaustion, and sit on the curb, in front of a mutual fund office, dejected with his chin between his palms.

Then, imagine Alexander the Great strolling by, again, and asking him what he would like. The odds may well be, that this time, Diogenes would probably respond with, "Get me some Prozac fast". Some might even speculate that possibly, he would also contemplate suicide."

Pursuit of Symptoms Over Causes may be a.k.a. the "band-aid or cover-up syndrome," which is very prevalent as a perceived anti-symptom silver bullet notion of instant, although brief, relief and/or gratification without affecting the cause. The goal of this syndrome is an attempt to "instantly annihilate the symptom, no matter what." It is also choosing denial of our choices, i.e., irresponsibility.

It may seem to some that a typical, but significant, consequence of symptom pursuit, or rather persecution, is the resulting creation of additional even if different symptoms not unlike a self-perpetuating ripple effect. In the meantime, the original symptom may at best be only temporarily held at bay. Had Hercules suffered from the band-aid syndrome, he would be still hacking away at Hydra's heads while being treated for acute tennis elbow with steroids.

Pursuit and Worship of Symbolism Over Substance is typically expressed by "that was a great and commendable deed or performance, but unfortunately it was not politically correct," or conversely, "it was a disastrous and shameful deed or performance, but fortunately it was politically correct." We continuously hear or observe this ultimate and canonized oxymoron in one form or another, and which is seemingly just as "acceptable" as a modern version of the *"Emperor's new clothes."* Embracing the oxymoron always leads to self-contradiction and internal conflict.

If one keeps selecting the sizzle over the steak, one may eventually starve. Maybe, some need to be reminded, at times, by the old lady of the burger commercial who said, *"Where is the beef?"* The old saying of *"The frock does not the monk make"* is right on.

The media reporting on the recent, huge, corporate scandals and the resulting disasters, commented that often the related CEOs had been previously elevated to rock star status by their directors, shareholders, the financial world, and, of course, the media. Apparently, they are all participating joyously at the Emperor's New Clothes game. Obviously, all this awe was aimed solely at the title/position and repute (which according to Goethe is nothing), i.e., the monk's frock.

When the sizzle sizzled off, everybody held an empty bag, or more appropriately an empty till. The media commented that some corporations may be choosing "repute" over talent.

Clemanceau, who took the reins during World War I in France, and shaped its military into a victorious force, commented on some general officers, *"It takes more than a hat of gold braids to turn an imbecile into an intelligent man."*

Someone once said that,

"Success is what everybody and his brother think you have accomplished. Achievement is what You know You have accomplished."

On this basis, success may be the symbolism, and achievement the substance. Pursuit of symbolism reminds one of an explorer lost in the Sahara and dying of thirst, who suddenly perceives an oasis on the shores of a cool lake and rushes with all his energy towards it, only to see it disappear after a few steps. Symbolism without substance is but a MIRAGE. Choosing symbolism over substance may be a rationalization (lie) designed to fool others, as well as one's self, the ultimate irresponsibility. Preconception is also an insidious form of symbolism over substance.

Lemming Syndrome is simply the old "me too regardless" game. Anecdotally, when one of these sub-arctic rodents dives in the frigid waters, then the others follow and also turn into Popsicles.

Starting in the 1990s, the odd acquisition-merger, IPO, creative accounting, etc., turned into an epidemic and spread faster than venereal disease. The resulting numerous and tragic debacles suffered by corporations, financial, and investment institutions, etc., may bear some resemblance to lemmings racing for the terminal dip in the icy waters, while telling themselves they are just being competitive.

The Lemming Syndrome is not restricted to the business world. It is present in every aspect of everyday life, and whenever we choose to pretend that the choice was already made for us by others, and we have but to follow, we then try to believe that we do not have to think, choose, or take responsibility. The official battle hymn of the lemmings was probably composed during the Clinton impeachment process.

"They all do it or everybody does it." And, "it" must therefore be ok.

The consequence of the attempt to relinquish our Free Will/Power of Choice is but the irresponsibility of self-deception. It consists of just rationalizing that, since the choice has been made by others, it must be ok and, therefore, we do not have to think and choose for ourselves. Being reminded that each one of us is unique, and that One-Size-Fits-All is but an oxymoronic myth, and the fact no one can make the choice for us but us, may prove helpful in choosing not to share icy waters with the lemmings. Some may conclude that there is no greater or more effective promoter of the Lemming Syndrome than the Advertising Media. Possibly it is the nuclear weapon of their arsenal or their Holy Grail depending on the point of view.

The Goal Justifies the Means may be valid for some in some instances, **provided** that the means does not replace or alter the goal. Otherwise it may be only a landmark rationalization attempting to fool one's self as well as others. Such a rationalization can be confusing, and may eventually lead to the following:

"The MEANS becomes the GOAL, and the GOAL becomes (the sustaining of) the MEANS" resulting in a self-perpetuating vicious circle of self-deception as well as that of others.

Historically, this has been the mainstay currency of despots and tyrants while they contemplated the sword of Damocles.

5 - CHOOSING TO BE IN CHARGE OF YOURSELF

Given who we are, being in charge of ourselves is simple, natural, powerful, safe, joyous, and just plain common sense. Or conversely, self destructive to the point of masochism, if we choose to deny who we are and our Free Will/Power of Choice. Simply put the law of Cause and Effect is always on the job.

Being who we are consists of the following:

- Each one of us is unique.

- We are all endowed with the absolute Free Will/Power of Choice.

- We are all equal.

- We all have equal opportunity.

The Universal law of Cause and Effect, through our Free Will/Power of Choice empowers our thoughts, words, and deeds, to create "causes" and their consequent "effects" too. Being mindful of the law of Cause and Effect, i.e., responsible, when we use our Free Will/Power of Choice will provide us with all the freedom we can handle.

Being in charge of ourselves is really a piece of cake if we choose to see it for what it is, just our inherent and absolute Free Will/Power of Choice over our own individual choices. You cannot choose for someone else without their consent, and their consent would make it their choice. In the same way, no one can choose for you without your consent, and your consent would make it your choice. Therefore, choosing to be in charge of anyone else's choices without their consent, or allowing somebody else to be in charge of your choices without your consent is absolutely impossible in both cases, and by refuting the impossible, you would in effect be choosing to fool yourself.

Being in Charge of Yourself may be supportive of the *"why do it the hard way, if you can do it the easy way"* philosophy (it would seem that it is UBB's philosophy as well.), versus the masochistic philosophy of *"why do it the easy way, if you can do it the hard way."*

Once the "easy way" is chosen, one may say good-bye to self-contradiction, internal conflict and fear, all the ingredients of that lethal cocktail, which is addictive to masochists and is called STRESS. Some may conclude that besides attempts at self-deception, by and large, the main source of self-contradiction and internal conflict is the possible clash between our very own thoughts-ideas-opinions and those of others, which we might have at one time or another erroneously adopted as our own.

Simply put, it is just a matter of acknowledging that you are the author of all your choices, both those you choose with responsibility and those you choose irresponsibly.

Dr. Wayne Dyer, the popular author and lecturer, uses the song, *"Row, row your boat,"* as a parable of life's reality, i.e., all you have to do is row your boat easily downstream while enjoying the experience, without trying to row someone else's boat, or pretending to allow someone else to row yours. That may be truly the "easy way."

Some may have observed that from cradle to grave non-stop, we are presented with fresh choices to choose at every instant. It is truly a *"l'embarras du choix"* situation.

Choice is, and has been, and will always be, yours and yours alone, and that puts you in charge, that is if you choose to be in charge.

Some may consider Freedom as the ultimate bonus of Being In Charge of one's self. Epictetus the first century AD philosopher concurred wholeheartedly saying,

"No man is free who is not master of himself."

When in charge of one's self, one may experience an empowering and exhilarating "beingness," in total liberty.

6 - CHOOSING TO BE IN CHARGE OF YOUR HEALTH... NOBODY ELSE CAN

You can buy all the healthcare in the world you can afford, and then some. But you *cannot buy health at any price, anywhere, anytime*, for the simple reason that you are its sole architect, and only you can create your own health should you so choose. It is part of our inherent and absolute Free Will/Power of Choice. This is how we were designed from the get go by the Big Bang, and within us reside the "specs" of our design, as well the designer's (UBB's) "maintenance manual." However, like all architects in charge you may "subcontract" here and there if and when you choose to.

Health is, indeed, so much more than wealth, *it is everything*.

Ancient Greek philosophers and physicians promoted the Healthy Mind in a Healthy Body concept. Modern scientists, more and more in agreement with the ancient Greeks, keep reconfirming that mental stress is hazardous to your physical and mental health. According to recent medical findings, mental stress also devastates our inherently invincible autoimmune system, i.e., our very own "homeland security organization," which is invincible, though only as long as we choose, not to overwhelm it.

During the dark ages in Europe, when the Abbassid dynasty was flourishing from Gibraltar to India, its physicians and philosophers concluded that, *"If you have health, you have hope, if you have hope, you have everything."*

The unhealthiest choice one can make is to deny ownership of one's health or relegating it to others and, therefore, denying responsibility for one's health. That would be tantamount to navigating your health's "Jeep" through the Rubicon Trail blindfolded, while asking and receiving directions and instructions from third parties over a cell phone. At best, such a scenario is literally a case of the blind leading the blind to certain disaster.

7 - WHAT HEALTH? WHERE?

Some of those who may choose the Yogi Berra approach of, *"You can sometimes see a lot just by looking,"* and observe the status of our collective health, may come up with the question of "What Health, Where?" without even being shocked. Because by now, it may have become part of the *"c'est la vie,"* or the "it happens to everybody" routine, and consequently, all our health problems may appear as inherent and natural and should, therefore, be suffered stoically and heroically, until we are parted with both wallet and life but only after suffering first.

We are daily and ever increasingly deluged with human health related information emanating from all kinds of media news, announcements by the scientific and medical communities, declarations, and/or measures by government agencies, various publications, and personal experiences, as well as those of family and acquaintances. Many are even included frequently in scenarios of the entertainment industry.

This ocean of information is quite alarming and confusing to say the least. One only has to observe the ever increasing carnage of cancer, heart disease, circulatory diseases of all kinds, respiratory diseases, diabetes, etc., etc., and the great plethora of diseases due to weakened dilapidated autoimmune systems.

A ten-year study, of about eight hundred older men

and women by the Rush University Medical Centre in Chicago, concluded that Diabetes increased the risk of developing Alzheimer's disease. A similar study in Europe reached parallel conclusions. It is estimated that about 18 Million Americans are afflicted with Diabetes, and according to the government about 41 Million Americans are in a pre-Diabetes mode, i.e., high blood sugar. Being overweight, and even more so, Obesity has been known to be a prime generator of Diabetes. Diabetes, besides Alzheimer's, it is also known to promote heart disease, circulatory diseases, kidney failure, etc., etc., and more recently it has been reported that it also substantially increases the risk of colon cancer. All this might look to some like a sinister domino effect within an ongoing vicious circle.

The latest icing on the cake is Obesity, at alleged epidemic proportions affecting all age groups, and which the medical establishment contends also gives birth to several of the above-mentioned diseases.

Consequently, it is tragically sad when the medical community feels compelled to start recommending that people should have regular, comprehensive heart check-ups starting as early as age twenty. High school, college, and professional young athletes, suffer heart failures more and more. Remember Darryl Kile of the Cardinals?

Another recommendation is that even pre-school children have to be watched for obesity, diabetes, asthma, and allergies. A more recent study in Ohio indicated that extremely obese youngsters can have heart abnormalities that puts them at serious risk of heart attacks. To top it all, a recent medical survey revealed that so far at least forty-seven of all the antidepressant drugs used by adults are now being prescribed to children. It practically sounds Biblical: *"The sins of the fathers...,"* etc.

At the same time, we are being informed that we never had it so good, allegedly because our life span has increased thanks to the never ending heroic scientific advances that keep us "alive and healthy." Meanwhile, according to the information Tsunami that hits us daily, it would seem that we are sick sooner, longer, and that we have multiple diseases simultaneously, which are frequently chronic, and that we might need a supersonic laptop with a large, pizza-sized hard disk just to sort out the plethora of medications, tests, diets, and supplements we supposedly have to take daily. While all this is taking place, we may be going broke at the same time as Medicare and Medicaid, and that does not include the additional privilege of personal suffering, stress, and/or even depression.

King Tut has been around for thousands of years. Some of us have even seen him in his native country or during his tours around the world. If only his physicians had access to today's "advanced" medical techniques and pills (probably needing as many slaves to feed him all the pills as those who built Great Pyramid), hi-tech plumbing and wiring hook-ups, and spare parts, he probably would be winking at us today. However, it is rather doubtful he would be enjoying his gold and his hunting chariots along with his "longevity." Martial, the first century AD Roman poet, was quite unequivocal when he stated, *"Life Is Not Living, But Living In Health"* (*non est vivere sed vaslere vita est*). Evidently, Martial was not a fan of the oxymoron.

Since we are told that we never had it so good, then disease and all its consequences may be taken for granted, taken as not only inevitable, but acceptable, a mere routine part of *"c'est la vie."* One major catchall scapegoat for the sorry state of our health is AGEING. "The more you age the sicker and more incapacitated you must get and the more medication you must take." This fearsome myth could seem to some, as tantamount to being sentenced to be buried alive, and tortured till the last breath. This myth too, was not part of "our Big Bang design specs," unless we choose it to be. As for those who might choose the myth, they may in vain chase till the end the mirage of health, let alone Ponce de Leon's fountain of youth.

According to Oliver Wendell Holmes, *"To be seventy years young is sometimes far more cheerful than to be forty years old."* It just sounds like a matter of choice again.

An alleged biology experiment comes to mind where biologists threw a live frog in a pot of boiling water, and the frog, with a lightning fast reflex action, jumped out instantly. They then threw the frog in a pot of cool water which they proceeded to heat slowly till it boiled. The frog never jumped out, and kept treading water complacently till it became soup du jour. The message of this experiment is that deteriorating conditions, if gradual, may become to some, tolerable and acceptable culminating in total and final complacency or even

46

"crutch dependency" till the bitter end.

At the same time, we are literally overwhelmed or rather force fed via the universal news/information media, the advertising media, books lectures, research findings, studies, statistics, scientific declarations, movies, TV shows et., etc., that there is allegedly always underway a colossal united effort to help us battle disease with everything our modern world has at its disposal.

This gigantic effort for the salvation of our health seems to be flooding us daily with recommendations, some contradictory almost immediately, and some upon further notice, later, and ditto for both side effects and after effects. They all have one thing in common though, the myth of One-Size-Fits-All.

There are millions if not billions of such recommendations floating around, but let's call them simply a myriad of recommendations, which consist of the following:

- Myriad of supplements and herbs.

- Myriad of special foods and beverages.

- Myriad of recommended foods and beverages.

- Myriad of foods and beverages to be avoided.

- Myriad of diets.

- Myriad of exercise and fitness systems.

- Myriad of non prescription drugs.

- Myriad of prescription drugs.

- Myriad tests.

- Myriad check-ups.

- Myriad vaccines.

- Myriad medical procedures and surgical interventions.

The list could go on and on, since these are just the highlights. Possibly, one of the underlying messages that all these recommendations may be conveying, is one of intimidation implying that "since they work for everybody else," if you do not follow them, then the consequences are suffering and possibly even death, which is a variant of the "if you don't go to church and confession every day, you will roast in hell forever."

Should one choose to follow only some, and not all the recommendations floating out there, one may have need of IBM's *Deep Blue,* the chess savvy computer that battled Gary Kasparov, the Russian world chess champion. It was not a mere laptop; it resembled the *Borg* spaceship that abducted Captain Jean-Luc Picard.

The *Deep Blue* would probably have to be active around the clock non-stop, just to comply with all the instructions and recommendations. What this could mean to one's lifestyle is best left to one's imagination. It is likely that twenty-four hours a day would not be enough for anyone to merely attempt to comply, let alone do something else as well. Some of those who may not "fully comply," might compensate for their guilt by rewarding themselves with ample additional stress and fear. To some, adherence to all the myriad dos and don'ts has degenerated to something more than "keeping up with the Joneses." It has practically become a sort of a "heroic" status symbol, as well as a sign of "stoic" pride.

It is probably quite conceivable that eventually in the name of "newer improved health and longer life," the scientific and healthcare establishments may decide to promote and heavily advertise recommendations and pills to regulate even our sympathetic nervous system, and then IBM's *Deep Blue* will no longer be able to cope. Our sympathetic nervous system is the miracle that automatically manages billions of processes in our bodies (most of which we are not aware of) non-stop, which enable us to live and function. These processes include also simpler things like blinking, yawning, and hair and nail growth, etc.

Just picture TV ads promoting a pill, which pretends to help one regulate blinking speed in the name of possibly preventing cataracts, glaucoma, and blindness as one grows older, or a pill to enhance the quality and frequency of yawning at specific times in order to improve your attention span, or yet another pill to slow toenail growth in order to prevent bunions, etc., etc. Possibly, even Jules Verne, the fellow who came up with Captain Nemo well over a century ago would not be able to keep up with all the promoters' "newer" potential scenarios for dispensing more pills.

All of which would have, supposedly, been preceded by appropriate research, studies, statistics, and then by finally securing FDA approval, with the latter meaning that it will probably not kill you over the weekend. Even arsenic did not kill Napoleon over a weekend; it took years of agony. Pending, of course, would be the inevitable and never-ending side and after effects and recall lists to be published later. Sound familiar? All of which probably, may eventually shoot health care costs past the GDP.

Research statistics, like all other statistics, may merely represent the "right arithmetic with the wrong numbers" let alone the insidious propagation of the One-Size-Fits-All myth, thus, once again ignoring our individual inherent uniqueness, or, as per Yogi, it's *"déjà vu all over again"* time...once again.

It is never too late for one to leap forward into the healthy life that one was designed and destined for, compliments of the Big Bang, provided of course one chooses to do so. The first step is to remember that one can choose to be in charge of one's self. The second step, once in charge of one's self, is that one may then choose to be in charge of one's health, and then the rest may very well be a piece of cake.

Dr. Andrew Weil, the popular author and lecturer on human health, seems to be of the opinion that the human body is designed to be able to take care of itself about eighty percent of the time, unless it is overwhelmed in its efforts to do so. Guess who does most of the overwhelming. If you guessed right, then you guessed it is up to You or Us to choose to give our health a fighting chance. As for the other twenty percent, e.g., a broken limb from a car accident, an appendectomy, etc., we may as the chief architect of our own health, subcontract for a direct medical intervention or health care services. Dr. Weil's apparent message is to cut our bodies some slack and give our health a break, at least most of the time.

Medical science has reported lately, that through a recent breakthrough in medical technology, it has proven that heart cells do regenerate after all and, therefore, may promote healing when the heart is damaged. Formerly, it was held that heart cells did not regenerate, and, therefore, an injury resulted in "dead" scar tissue. To Witch Doctors around the world, this latest scientific "Eureka" has been for millennia a *"déjà vu all over again."* Dr. Weil would probably agree with this latter day "Eureka." Why not? After all, we are the Big Bang's GUP (Gizmo of Ultimate Perfection).

8 - THE SYMPTOM SUPPRESSION JIHAD

The pursuit-of-symptoms-versus-causes philosophy seems to prevail also in our health care approach. It would seem that for some, the appearance of some physical discomfort, pain, or concerns for any other body symptoms, are inevitable if not "natural." A frequent reaction is that science or somebody has something to "take care of it," whatever "it" is, and lets do it pronto and think nothing of it. Such a scenario could possibly be expressed in this manner, "give me the right silver bullet for assured and instant gratification and don't bother me with the details or the consequences," and the response frequently is the same as in the service and retail industries: "what the customer/patient wants, the customer/patient gets." This scenario may, therefore, ignore both causes of the symptoms as well as the side effects and/or after effects of the silver bullet itself. Over time, a culture of pursuing the symptoms all the time and at all costs seems to have taken hold on both healthcare givers and healthcare recipients. Such a culture alleges a "scientific silver bullet" assuring instant gratification perceived or otherwise no matter the consequences, which may best be described by the notorious expression of Louis XIV of France, *"Après moi, le déluge."*

By and large causes of "unhealth" may be due to "Aristotelian Immoderation," i.e., all kinds of excesses or imbalances, which may eventually succeed in overwhelming health. Just one example of the countless excesses is the repeated alert of antibiotic overuse. According to the medical establishment, this universal overuse of antibiotics has already produced some disastrous results that potentially can be amplified further. Therefore, focusing on symptoms, while ignoring the causes, may result in a perpetual treatment of symptoms that can even create dependency, while the causes may well develop further, evolve or amplify their symptoms and maybe even create new ones. Simultaneously, the symptom treatment itself could, very well over time, create new causes with their very own set of symptoms, and on and on, like a never ending combination of ripple and domino effects.

Such a conclusion would not seem too far fetched, if one tunes in to the never ending daily updates on human health related information emanating from all kinds of news media, announcements by the scientific community, declarations, and/or measures by government agencies, personal experiences, as well as those of family members and acquaintances. Those seeking awareness, and/or confirmation of the above, can obtain it daily in copious amounts, simply by tuning in on the news provided by the major networks, not to mention the print media.

Adding fuel to the fire is the seemingly concerted promotion, and all kinds of advertising, of symptom prevention efforts. This idea may be additionally promoted by implying something like: "If you do not currently share the same affliction or suffering with Tom, Dick, and Harry, in time you will, as it eventually but inevitably happens to everybody, so you better act now by adopting this treatment this minute." The old myth of One-Size-Fits-All strikes again. Maybe not all, but some may seem quite eager to comply with such suggestions anyway.

It is amazing what intimidation can accomplish, and it is even used to influence our drinking habits. We have been relentlessly bombarded with the idea that "dehydration can provoke all kinds of health problems, and we are all dehydrated and we do not even know it," and according to "research findings," we should drink certain quantities of water at certain intervals, "or else." That implies that people never experienced the sensation of thirst, or should ignore it simply because they are being told to. End result is the comic sight of some people "mechanically" sipping water all day whether they feel like it or not while carrying around plastic bottles of commercially bottled water. Only a formal survey can determine who are currently the majority, water bottle haulers, or cell phone haulers. Now that cell phone manufacturers include digital cameras in the cell phones, the next step is probably to include a "digital water reservoir." Maybe in this era of globalisation and merger mania this could become reality if Motorola and Evian were to merge.

Naturally succeeding studies dispute the previously recommended number of bottles to be consumed or when and how. The UBB is obviously a fan of the KISS principle. The deal being that whenever our body needs to be hydrated, our thirst sensation would kick in automatically, and then we would drink until the thirst sensation subsided, till the next time.

Dr. Arthur Siegel who is a Harvard University professor as well as Chief of Internal Medicine at the McLean Hospital in Belmont, Mass would seem to concur at least as far as those engaged in intense exercise such as running marathons are concerned. According to Dr. Siegel, a marathon runner himself one of the risks of sudden death in running marathons or due to any intense physical activity for that matter is hyponatremia, i.e. "overhydration". Apparently, in recent years, healthy, young and older marathon runners have died participating in marathons, of hyponatremia, or "H_2O Overdose". Those who follow the faddish folkloric recommendation to drink lots of water particularly during physical activity may be risking their lives. Dr. Siegel suggests drinking only when thirsty will prevent hyponatremia. Simply put drink only when you feel thirsty, that is how we are built. just follow the signs your body gives you. That said, however, if you were crossing the Sahara on a pair of sneakers, carrying a bottle or two of water might not be such a bad idea. Reportedly, it would seem that most of the time regular tap water was at least as safe as bottled water, and in most cases "tastier."

Meanwhile, back at the ranch, the following with all their ramifications, seemingly continued to be amplified almost geometrically:

- Health and resulting life quality deterioration.

- Costs of health care.

- Pursuit of the symptom silver bullet mirage.

- Proliferation of drug manufacturers and health givers heavy advertising.

The medical and pharmaceutical establishments are working at a feverish pitch for newer, bigger, better weapons to treat symptoms and the myriad of resulting, anticipated or not, side and/or after effects. Research and experimentation "is on overtime," and so is the backlogged FDA.

As reported daily in the news of at least the major networks, there are many, many drugs, treatments, supplements, etc., and the benefits of which are at one time or another disproved and potentially harmful and therefore "recalled," not to mention their, to date, known side effects. One may again wonder if FDA approval is but some kind of assurance that it will not kill you over the weekend. It might seem at times that more time and effort is expended to analyse and catalogue symptoms, than on cause investigation and research.

Automobiles, particularly those previewed in car shows or Formula-1 vehicles, are becoming more and more sophisticated and hi-tech, and are all equipped with countless sensors to alert the driver about a multitude of functions and situations of concern. There may be some drivers around who, when they see something light up on the dashboard, find that all they want to do is eliminate it by disconnecting a wire or covering it up with duct tape (not necessarily the kind recommended by Homeland Security) and then just drive on. There are, of course, folks who will even provide assistance to such drivers, by disconnecting the wires or selling them duct tape and even applying for them the duct tape.

Surprise, surprise, such drivers as those in this parable are probably the biggest repeat customers of the car towing industry, as well as prime suppliers to junkyards.

News flash: The human body is far more complex and sophisticated than the automobile. It is indeed a mini-Universe in itself. Yet some may treat it like the above mentioned drivers treat their cars, and if that treatment causes even more light-ups, then more wires might be pulled, more duct tape and band-aids used, etc., on and on, producing an everlasting combination ripple and domino effects.

In comparison, chopping off Hydra's heads without Hercules may be less frustrating and more productive. Speaking of Hercules, the Zeus Club members may be proud to know that Hera a.k.a. Mrs. Zeus, who never was his mother, proved through DNA testing that Zeus is indeed his dad.Subject, of course, to confirmation by the FBI labs.

At times, extensive TV ads promoting certain indigestion or heartburn remedies, show people devouring with great gusto some "culturally correct" (but possibly suspect) fast foods, followed by lots of discomfort, followed by the "miraculous" remedy coming to the rescue by providing instant relief. Naturally, this was just one rough interpretation of some commercials. Imagine something similar and parallel about an automotive ad. The ad would show a car running repeatedly over spike boards (like those used by police in roadblocks or by some parking lots) and the resulting flat tires. Then, a spray can of "IFM" (Instant Flat Miracle) would appear and spray the tires, and instantly, everything is back to normal. The ad closes with, *"now you can run over your favourite spike board all you want without discomfort or worry, IFM is on guard for thee."* Naturally, the side and after effects of the spray on the tire compound would be printed on the back label in very, very small print. Later, there will of course be "newer, improved" versions of "IFM" let alone what the competition may come up with. Eventually, the "IFM" and the spike board manufacturers may merge together to keep producing newer improved sprays and newer more effective (damaging) spike boards, "so everybody can live happily ever after." Hopefully, not many would keep looking for spike boards to drive over. Unfortunately, however, but equally likely and knowingly, some may keep on ingesting what brings on the indigestion and/or heartburn in the first place. Some may rationalize it as being par for the course, and then reach for the well advertised "band-aid" pill. By observing the state of human health around us, it may seem that unlike the old classic AVIS commercial, the harder we try the "behinder" we get.

As a result of the Symptom Suppression Jihad, more and more and newer improved "band-aids" are concocted all the time. Some of them are to be taken for life, almost all of them have side and/or after effects known or not as yet, and some have effects with immediate and devastating results. At times, some methods of symptom relief are stopped or reversed way after the fact or when it is already too late. This process at times seems to resemble a stab in the dark kind of trial and error experimentation. Yet, at times it might seem rationalized and even institutionalized, as just part of science and technology waging a valiant all out war against disease, while attempting to prolong life. Sort of a Russian roulette for a "noble" cause. Maybe, at best, it is but a risky exercise in futility anyway, as the One-Size-Fits-All concept does not work since we are each unique, and also because of the focus on symptoms rather than causes. The Symptom Suppression Jihad is conceivably supported by many of those who may have adopted or are addicted to a "just hand me the band-aid this minute and don't bother me with the details" mentality. For validation just dip daily into the overflowing rivers of published and broadcast health related information surrounding us.

This extensive experimentation relentlessly "utilizes" human beings as guinea pigs, all in the name of healing, longevity, and quality of life improvement. Some people seem to quite willingly subject themselves to "experiments" that may prove worse than the disease. Maybe, if the infamous Dr. Mengele, and his "boys from Brazil", had stumbled into such an environment of practically unlimited guinea pig volunteers, they would have possibly thought they had reached the "Volunteer Guinea Pig Hog Heaven" and had endless "fun," non-stop and with impunity.

The irony is that many groups protest and fight to keep animals from being used as "guinea pigs," and do not seem to say a word about human beings where the experimentation (although it is often called the latest medical breakthrough) is happening on a much larger scale. It would require endless volumes to list the trial and error "side and/or after effects" already on record, not to mention that there are additions daily. Just remember, not the Alamo this time, but the THALIDOMIDE tragedies of the past.

In spite of the prevailing symptom pursuit, and One-Size-Fits-All cultures, it may be quite hard to imagine that a physician or a healthcare provider is deliberately trampling all over the Hippocratic ethics. On the other hand one may ask, could this culture exist without the willing and sometimes eager participation of the healthcare recipients themselves.

A recently deciphered ancient Babylonian (definitely pre-Saddam) tablet relating to human health stated that,

"The best physician is always the physician who talks the most with his patient." It may be a safe bet that this patient-physician discussion was not about the "proliferation of arms of mass destruction in the region" (even though it could have been the "right neighbourhood"). The dialogue may have rather been a form of extensive debriefing, maybe even as intense as that of Al Qaeda's captured top lieutenant, Khalid Sheikh Mohammed.

Probably the "best" Babylonian physician, recognized and acknowledged, that each patient was unique, and that he had to gather as many of the equally unique clues as possible in trying to determine probable causes and the resulting symptoms of discomfort. To that end, he needed the patient's experiences and interpretations, his lifestyle, habits, etc., almost similar to a homicide investigation at the crime scene. The physician would then analyze the input, pick out facts, and compare them with his own knowledge and experience, before proceeding with treatment. Basically trying to alter, diminish, or eliminate anything that might be attempting to overwhelm the body and mind system, and/or trying to assist the system ("repair itself as designed") by stopping and/or reversing any "overwhelming." Just as Dr. Andrew Weil has stated on Larry King,

"You want to facilitate healing, not prevent it."

Maybe the Babylonian physicians had recognized that indeed One-Size-DOES NOT-Fit-All and, therefore, the need to customize the "facilitating" assistance provided to each patient.

A cursory observation may reveal, that most likely, this may not be happening nowadays. The health care system as set up, although well intentioned, may well be most of the time incapable of expending such an effort with the patient due to time, financial, and other constraints. On the other hand, in some cases, a Babylonian style of patient debriefing might even be unfeasible, as some people may not be aware of, or even interested in their mind-body system, let alone how it functions, reacts, etc. Their main interest possibly being only in something to eliminate the symptom(s) of discomfort, and if possible, temporarily alleviate any resulting worries and fears they might have. They are probably happiest with the physician with fastest draw of the pen to prescribe "instant relief pills," and maybe some tests that will either alleviate fears or add some more pills at the very least, no questions asked. Such patients could not provide the physician with any helpful clues beyond describing the "unbearable" discomfort of their symptoms if their life depended on it. They may, however, relate (conversationally, at least) quite well to the diseases of others as described by the news and advertising media and other sources, to the point of taking ownership of the diseases, and asking for the prevailing typical One-Size-Fits-All treatment any way if only as a preventive measure. Ben Franklin, who probably had not read the Babylonian tablet, said, *"He's the best physician that knows the worthlessness of the most medicines."*

Inherently, some symptom suppressing treatments (as well as their side and/or after effects) are of long duration, if not lifelong, which brings to mind this old saying: "Drop by drop, a drop of water may eventually pierce granite."

Just picture what chronic medication may accomplish, while remembering that we are not made out of granite. Even arsenic in small enough quantities can take many years of suffering till it kills. Just ask Napoleon, he was not made out of granite either. France recognized recently the authentic accuracy of the book *The Murder of Napoleon* and adopted its findings as historical fact, i.e., that Napoleon had indeed been slowly and deliberately poisoned over many years with arsenic. Socrates on the other hand was very fortunate to just sip hemlock once. The contents of the book remind one of Sherlock Holmes, and his sometime latest rival "CSI : Miami" as they also unmask the murderers. It took tremendous research, and collection of information, plus twenty years of brilliant detection effort by the Swedish doctor Sten Forshufvud, a prominent poison expert, capped by modern forensic medicine, and confirmed by the FBI labs.

The suffering of Napoleon, as described in detail in the various journals of the members of his entourage in St. Helena, may convey images of a slow motion crucifixion. Some may identify those various symptoms with those that are apparent today through a variety of mainly chronic causes Then, as today, symptoms were pursued instead of the cause, except that Napoleon's physician was far more limited. Sir Arthur Conan Doyle was a dentist, and so was Dr. Sten Forshufvud. Arthur's hobby was the study of tobaccos; Sten's hobby was the study of poisons. They were both dentists and both had chemistry related hobbies, and both were masters of detection, coincidence?

Consequently, France gratefully awarded Ben Weider, the author of the book, the Legion d'Honneur medal, recognizing at the same time that he is one of the most dedicated, if not the most dedicated expert and fan of Napoleon, and owns one of the most extensive private collections of Napoleonic memorabilia coveted even by the land of freedom fries. He is also a member of the Order of Canada. But, most importantly, Ben is a genuine Mensch. Those in need of confirmation of the latter, may contact the "Governator" of California (a.k.a. the terminator of "girlie-men"). Ben and his brother Joe recognized and appreciated Arnie's talents the moment he arrived from the land of the Blue Danube. The Brits also owe Ben some gratitude, as he exonerated them. Since Napoleon's death, the French and practically everybody else pointed the rumour finger at the Brits, i.e., a "007" on the island had done Napoleon in.

It would take less than a week's (any week, all the time) TV news and ads to acknowledge and appreciate the sad state of our collective health and validate, possibly, all of the above. It might even conjure images of a rabid dog desperately chasing its tail non-stop, while the unfortunate outcome appears certain. Attacking the cause of disease holistically can be compared to D-Day in Normandy, while attacking the symptom would be like the Dieppe Raid at best. Regardless of any amount of Dieppe Raids, Europe might still be occupied today, i.e., a chronic occupation. Some may conclude that the Symptom Suppression Jihad may very well be the primary and major contributor of chronic disease. Evidently, if the cause of the disease is not addressed, it will not go away and its stay will become chronic and even permanent

A national daily publication reported that chronic diseases in the US alone seemed to affect at least 125 million people, and cost over 500 billion dollars in 2003. This was news that was followed later by the declaration of Tommy Thomson Secretary of Health and Human Services that there are over 125 million Americans afflicted with chronic disease and that seventy-five percent of the 1.5 TRILLION dollars in health care costs are spent on chronic diseases, He then went on to say that a lot can be prevented with appropriate nutrition and physical activity accompanied by no smoking, and some funds saved could then be diverted to unavoidable health emergencies. In a nutshell, he too seems to be recommending pursuit of the cause over the chronic pursuit of symptoms.

Not too long ago, a major national TV news network included in its morning program an interview with a physician regarding two sleeping pills just approved by the FDA, and available to the public. According to the physician, these latest "newer, better, improved" sleeping pills, to date, seem to promise less side effects, and as for after effects, it is probably still, too soon. The interviewer asked if the physician would take the pills. The physician replied, *"I am somewhat old fashioned, and I would rather hunt down the cause of insomnia, be it too much caffeine, too much alcohol, late dinner, inappropriate mattress, stressful worries, etc. Then I would attempt to deal with, the cause."* Was this physician just expressing faith in the good old "Physician heal thyself?" To some such an "old fashioned" physician might seem like a breath of fresh air while, on the other hand, others may consider the Symptom Suppression Jihadist physicians, as very "fashionable."

About the same time, a national daily publication reported on a recent study regarding increasing misdiagnosis related to MRIs. The study found that this was mainly due to over focusing on analyzing the

MRI results, and under focusing on clinical diagnosis. Could something parallel be happening with other tests? Some may conclude that the ancient Babylonian tablet seemed to also emphasize clinical diagnosis, since it recommended extensive dialogues between patient and physician.

Symptom pursuit without eliminating the cause, inherently promotes chronic medication, which renders the cause chronic as well, while chronic medication may also become chronic dependency. The difference with heroin dependency is that it is called drug addiction; they are both hazardous to one's health at the very least.

In the end, suppressing the symptom is just as futile and dangerous as:

"Killing the messenger and burying the message."

9 - THE LAB RAT SYNDROME

There are daily news barrages of technological breakthrough treatments, newer research findings, new recommendations, etc., focused mainly on symptoms and which is, eventually, at times, backed by heavy advertising. All this information, and/or these recommendations, are not restricted to medication, surgery, and other medical procedures, but also diets, foods, beverages (both modified, treated or not), supplements, exercises, lifestyles, etc. Invariably, if not inevitably, these recommendations have a historical tendency at times, to be reversed and the products recalled, and maybe even followed by severe health damage, suffering, and possibly even death. Then, there are published lists and these lists, which are lengthened daily, as reported by all media of possible side and after effects, which may appear to function simply on the basis of "buyer beware." This may be ok if one is buying a pair of sneakers, but not necessarily when one's health, welfare, and even life, are involved. Possibly, the myth of One-Size-Fits-All, and not heeding Aristotle's golden rule against excess, are important contributors to this situation.

It would appear that during the last two decades of the twentieth century, the nation's state of health has markedly deteriorated, while healthcare costs have increased substantially, suffering has amplified, and all of this continues at an ever-accelerating pace.

Awareness of the above can be obtained, confirmed, and maintained, daily through the news and advertising media, in addition to just observing life unfold around you.

Yet, there are ongoing declarations that, *"due to scientific advances, human health care quality has never been better, while quality of life has been enhanced and life expectancy extended."* The observant might find that this contradicts what is happening around us (if not to us), and that maybe these declarations add up to not much more than *"Enron's declared profits."* On the other hand, didn't the notorious Dr. Goebbels mumble that the more you repeat the biggest and most incredible lie, the more credible it becomes. Right up to the total collapse of Saddam's regime, his ubiquitous minister of information Mohammed Said al-Sahaf a.k.a. "Baghdad Bob" kept validating, again and again, Dr. Goebbels' doctrine about Iraqi victories. It finally took a live split TV screen to convince the Iraqi public he was lying, though many still continue to believe him.

It would seem at times, that healthcare givers may rationalize, that it is all done for the noble cause of advancing the science of saving lives at all costs (even a la King Tut), no matter the results. Could it be that it is just an endless pursuit of short-term Pyrrhic victories? At the same time, it would seem that some healthcare recipients may have rationalized the situation as an inevitable kismet that can be best countered with a stoic, if not heroic "grin and bear it" attitude, while automatically submitting to the "latest findings and recommendations" no questions asked, while some of the "lucky" suffering survivors may even end up broke and/or depressed. It may appear that in the name of health and preservation, some people have willingly turned themselves into lab rats in unprecedented numbers in this, a full three hundred and sixty degrees domino effect, which treats the symptom while the cause may keep on producing newer symptoms, and while at the same time symptom treatments may produce their own series of symptoms, as if each falling domino produces its own self-perpetuating ripple effect as well. Maybe the myth of the Lerne Hydra monster could be viewed as a fitting parable for this conundrum. If some find this incredible, they don't have to research much, because all they have to do is to keep track of the news and advertising media, which confirms it practically daily and with no likely end in sight.

The results may seem to some as an indication that this apparent all out scientific effort, in the name of health and longevity, is often but a stab in the dark and each stab opens its own Pandora's Box, which in turn would require its own set of stabs in the dark. Some may find that by comparison Russian roulette is but a game of bingo.

Such efforts seem to be generated at best by good intentions and/or wishful thinking and, at worse, by various selfish motives. The resulting paradox is that the healthcare suppliers for the most part act with the best intentions, while the healthcare recipients for the most part may silently accept the offered healthcare even when it produces the most tragic results, with the proverbial stiff upper lip. In other words, they may be taking it all for granted. Yet, as observed, some of the very same people may justifiably "cry murder," when some SUV manufacturers experiment with certain tires, that fall apart and the vehicles flip over. This phenomenon begs the question about whether experimentation with vehicles resulting in tragic outcomes is not ok, but experimentation with human health, at times with even more tragic results, is ok?

Could there be somewhere a parallel between some of those who endure silently the suffering of these trial and error symptom treatments, and the biology experiment where the frog kept swimming in that pot of water till it became soup du jour? Another possible parallel illustration could be the scene from H. G. Wells' *The Time Machine* movie (starring Rod Taylor), where the peaceful and beautiful people, the *Elois,* who had been conditioned to inevitably flock to the caves of the *Morloks* are devoured by these cannibals, who they viewed as their "benefactors," whenever a siren was activated.

What is equally remarkable is that some inflict the same trial and error symptom treatment on their beloved pets, by feeding them the same drugs they themselves use, including antidepressants, and with the same results one might add. Some may even remember Al Gore, during his 2000 presidential bid talking about Medicare, when he complained that his mother's arthritis medication cost so much more than the identical medication for her dog's arthritis.

Is it possible that some have wilfully become

gradually but perpetually the most compliant and disposable breed of lab rats? It would appear that the difference, between, humans and the rodents, is that the rodents never volunteer for lab rat duty. But then again who knows, they might well volunteer, if they were sufficiently exposed to TV and other ads. Following the latest government figures, which again prove that many people are leading unhealthy lives, Dan Blumenthal, chairman of community health and preventive medicine at Morehouse School of Medicine said, *"It's almost as if the elements are conspiring against us to lead unhealthy lifestyles."* He added, *"We are faced with a constant barrage of advertising on television about fast food. We live in a world where we are encouraged to drive more and walk less and spend more time in front of our televisions."*

A report published by a national daily publication seems to echo some of Dan Blumenthal's comments. Apparently, the number of Americans afflicted with osteoporosis multiplied by seven in the decade between 1993 and 2004. According to a Stanford University study, this substantial increase coincided with the introduction of non-hormonal osteoporosis medication. The previous hormonal therapy had lost popularity due to concerns linking them to cancer, heart disease, and other risks. Consequently, the Estrogen alternatives grew into a multi-billion industry annually boosted by heavy and wide advertising. Both Dr. Randall Stafford, who led the study, and Dr. Ethel Siris, head of the National Osteoporosis Foundation's science and research committee seem to have concluded that the "old standbys," calcium and vitamin D in one form or another, as well as exercising are contributors to osteoporosis prevention. *"Back to the Future,"* again.

As one may readily observe, the advertising barrage is limited neither to television or fast foods. It is everywhere and about everything, It can affect lifestyles and health or lack thereof, provided we choose to allow it. Should we choose to allow it, however, then who knows, maybe Saddam's ubiquitous and colorful ex- minister of information, Mohammed Said al-Sahaf a.k.a. "Baghdad Bob," might eventually land a top job on Madison Avenue. After all, he did a heck of a job promoting Saddam's victories over the coalition forces.

However, the information that is unleashed upon us daily seems to indicate that the apparent all out effort by healthcare suppliers and healthcare recipients, in the Symptom Suppression Jihad, is apparently Sisyphian, except for a short Pyrrhic victory here and there. This ongoing at all costs Jihad against symptoms may appear to some as being carried in the spirit of *"Après moi, le deluge."*

More recently, just like *"The Return of Dracula"* movies, Thalidomide is back as a treatment for symptoms other than morning sickness symptoms, accompanied with all kinds of side effects, or if you will "Collateral Damage" warnings, as for after effects, just keep posted. It may be only a matter of time, that for one reason or another, we might learn that Dracula struck again.

Since the Gulf war, and all subsequent conflicts,

miss-targeted and/or unintended destruction has been described in military parlance as "Collateral Damage", possibly because it might sound less "personal" and appear rather innocuous, or regrettably unavoidable if not accidental, as well as somewhat "politically correct." It has, however, never consoled the recipients (victims) of the Collateral Damage, or spared the military due or undue criticism and/or condemnation. The same thing, however, in healthcare parlance is called "Side and/or After Effects," and most seem to accept it without even a whimper, let alone criticism or condemnation, and probably, most, buy into it automatically, except for the occasional counterattack of the "tort virus" (mostly of the Class Action strain).

Imagine a label on the laser guided bombs used against Saddam, indicating "Radical Medication prescribed for terminal tyranny, and with Side and after effects listed on the other side." If the military adopted the medical parlance, i.e., Side/After Effects, they might be less criticized or condemned. On the other hand, if healthcare adopted the military parlance of Collateral Damage, then even the most devoted, well-intentioned, symptom Jihadists might slow down their frenzied quest for the mythical, symptom-slaying, silver bullet.

Some, when attacking their symptoms, may well want to consider their body as an ally and not an enemy, and even spare them any "friendly fire" attack as well as the "Collateral Damage."

Some may concur that the Human Being a.k.a. GUP (Gizmo of Ultimate Perfection) has been created marvellously perfect and autonomous, as a self-sustaining, self-regenerating, self-repairing creation, and is a little universe in its own right, simple and complex at the same time. However, given the present state of human health, it might sound like an oxymoron until our Free Will/Power of Choice is factored into the equation. This creation can be wondrously simple and efficient should we choose to allow it and assist it to function as designed by the Big Bang itself.

Could it be that healthcare efforts concentrating on symptom suppression are but attempts to second guess, mimic, or in futile duplication, or maybe even counteract and/or overwhelm, this marvellous creation without having even a glimpse of the "Big Picture" or the "Grand Perspective" if you will, let alone comprehend it. If this is indeed the case, it may be preferable to gain a greater understanding and appreciation of the Big Picture, i.e., the Big Bang's concept and design "specs" for humans, and assist it to do the perfect job it was designed to do, without second-guessing it or impeding it in any way. It may not only prove more effective, but also easier, simpler, satisfying, and last but not least healthier. It probably would work wonders for one's pocketbook as well.

Some may believe that reason and science can uncover everything and anything in the Big Bang's Universe heretofore unknown. The state of our health indicates we are a long way from such an achievement. Immanuel Kant, the eighteenth century German philosopher, more or less concluded that human beings are basically limited by their five senses and the resulting experiences no matter how reasoned, are not limitless, and may leave a lot unknown, which may never be known. Maybe Aristotle had a point when he said, *"The physician heals, Nature makes well."*

A Gallic version much later by Voltaire indicated that, *"Physicians distract the patients while Nature heals them."*

The impressive sort of cutting-edge scientific documentary movie *"What The Bleep Do We Know*?" aired in the summer of 2004. An equally impressive array of heavy-duty scientists contributed to this realization. The question posed by the title of the movie, as well as the movie content, may seem to jive with Immanuel Kant's position that we have limitations and there may be a lot we do not have a clue about and may never get one. Voltaire also shared similar thoughts which he expressed not as delicately as Kant *"Doctors are men who prescribe medicines of which they know little, to cure diseases of which they know less, in human beings of whom they know nothing"*.

The movie also seems to agree with Sophocles about the magnificently wonderful "GUP" a.k.a Human Being.

In the meantime, by exercising our Free Will/Power of Choice, and working hand in hand with the marvellous mind and body we were given, we might yet cease trying to overwhelm it, and quit behaving like aspiring lab rats and thus at least stop worrying about and coping with "Side Effects/Collateral Damage," etc.

10 - IT IS NOT ALL GREEK AFTER ALL

A healthy mind in a healthy body is what ancient Greek philosophers and physicians fervently maintained as a philosophy. But it is no longer "all Greek" to scientists. The most recent scientific findings of studies and research keep reconfirming the ancient Greek findings. In ancient Greece, mind meant much more than just a mass of grey, slimy matter, and they certainly included the intuition/feelings factor to say the least. Yogi Berra it seems also reached a similar parallel conclusion having said that, *"ninety percent of baseball is half mental."* Following up on Yogi's conclusions is Harvard University psychologist Steven Kosslyn, who made a name for himself with his work on the connection between mind and brain. He maintains that *"Body and mind are not as separate as they appear to be; not only does the state of the body affect the mind, but also vice versa."* This has not been translated back to Greek as yet. Adding fuel to the fire, by the end of 2003, a University of California (not of ancient Athens) study revealed that,

"Those who count their blessings are less vulnerable to disease."

The Six Key Self-Evident Factors affecting human health are:

- Everything Ingested.

- Everything Inhaled.

- Physical Activity.

- Lifestyle.

- State of Mind.

- Stress.   (It can be powerfully devastating and can affect the other five factors.)

Some of the effects of these Six key Factors may and can damage human health. Some treatments to repair the damage may also produce effects that may just as well at times amplify or multiply the damage. Basically, all effects are the consequences of choices made, as the Free Will/Power of Choice is incessantly exercised. It is nothing more than the Universal Law of Cause and Effect at work, just like the Universal Law of Gravity, which is also always there on the job.

In an effort to counteract the effects of these Six Key Factors of human health, , a veritable "Tower of Babel" founded on the One-Size-Fits-All myth and the Symptom Suppression Jihad seems to be in the process of being continuously and feverishly erected. It consists primarily of these often contradictory, rectified and at times hazardous myriad recommendations/ advice, once again, about the following:

- Myriad of supplements and herbs.

- Myriad of special foods and beverages.

- Myriad of recommended foods and beverages.

- Myriad of foods and beverages to be avoided.

- Myriad of diets.

- Myriad of exercise and fitness systems.

- Myriad of non prescription drugs.

- Myriad of prescription drugs.

- Myriad tests.

- Myriad check-ups.

- Myriad vaccines.

- Myriad medical procedures and surgical interventions.

"Building and demolition activities" on this modern Tower of Babel are incessant, while its scope is ever expanding, as demonstrated by the daily barrages of additional technological "breakthrough" treatments, "newer" research findings, new recommendations, etc., which are focused mainly on symptoms and frequently backed by heavy advertising. Exacerbating the situation, food companies are now emulating the pharmaceutical companies and are promoting their products directly to physicians, as well as enlisting them for direct promotions.

To some this Tower of Babel may appear to have appointed itself as the "sole" intermediary between people and their health and well-being. Some might even view it as a parallel to the high priesthood of ancient Egypt, who appointed themselves as salvation intermediaries between the people and their deities, through all kinds of rituals, dogmas, sacrifices, etc., and all done under the umbrella of the original and most formidable weapon of mass destruction, FEAR. If only FDR had been around at the time to remind the terrified Egyptians that, *"they had nothing to fear but fear itself."* Speaking of fear, some may have already experienced what La Fontaine said about fear a few centuries ago (and it was not one of his fables), which was that, *"From a distance it is something; and nearby it is nothing."*

These never-ending barrages of health related information emanate from all kinds of media news announcements by the scientific community, declarations and/or measures by government agencies, as well as from personal, family, and acquaintance's anecdotal experiences.

Complementing these is the ever expanding myriad of side and after effects reports, recalls, retractions, reversals, some of them are even catastrophic, either in the short or more often in the long term. Some even initiated by the myriad of recommendations in the first place. The all-encompassing oxymoron is the fact that all these myriad are based on the myth of One-Size-Fits-All. In retrospect, the confusion that reigned in the original Tower of Babel may have been as simple as riding a tricycle. Could it be that all of this is but a road leading from one excess to another? In which case, Aristotle would be having heartburn in his grave. If only somebody would show him how to "spell relief"...R-o-l-a-i-d-s.

Equally alarming are the alterations, additions, etc., of anything we ingest in the name of better, faster, easier, newer, more convenient, and allegedly healthier, or at least harmless. In retrospect, as proven time and again, they were often just proverbial stabs in the dark motivated mostly by the search for convenience, comfort, and efficiency, for either or both suppliers and consumers, but at times resulting in harmful side and/ or after effects. These, in turn, may be halted only to be replaced by more of the same.

In 2004, the University of Texas at Austin concluded a study of comparative analysis of fruit and vegetables (43 varieties) between current crops and those of 50 years ago. The findings indicated a significant and widespread decline in vitamins, minerals, and other nutrients. A previous, similar study in England reached parallel conclusions. It is suspected that modern farming methods may have something to do with it. Once more, it might seem that the "most convenient and efficient" (for whom?) farming methods are being selected no matter the results, i.e., side and after effects. Could it be that the proponents of the modern farming methods "inadvertently" triggered the vitamin, mineral, and nutrient supplements mega industry which is thriving like never before, or were they "visionaries" who then possibly "diversified" by heavily investing in it?

Although the study did not address a taste comparison of fruit and vegetables, some consumers might find today's crops, are substantially lacking in taste, to say the least.

However there does not seem to be any **consumer**

outrage, this perhaps being the result of the methodical and pervasive "dumbing down" of one's taste buds over the years.

The Texas study did not particularly address other kind of chemical treatments (e.g. for "looks and a longer shelf life") that the crops are subjected to by the time they arrive on the supermarket shelves. Is it again a case of symbolism over substance?

Some might have observed a parallel situation with the cut flowers of today, which look great and seem to last longer. Once upon time, a single rose would practically scent a whole apartment. Today, some could possibly stuff their nose with rose petals and either smell nothing or exclaim, "They sure don't smell like they used to." Again, a reminder that our senses are vital channels of communication between mind and body.

One may also wonder! what a similar study comparing "regular" crops with genetically modified crops 50 years from now would indicate?.

The repetitive destruction of tons and tons of e-coli contaminated hamburger ground beef, following consumer infections and even deaths, has been increasing. The meatpackers, backed by some scientific reports, recommended irradiation as the surest means to destroy the e-coli bacteria, allegedly, without any harm to humans. Yet other reports seem to warn that irradiation may indeed be harmful to humans. Some other reports seem to indicate that inadequate sanitation in the handling of meat was the source of contamination and it could be addressed effectively without irradiation, which still seems controversial as far as benefits versus harm, even though some foods are already being irradiated.

Could it be that irradiation requires less effort and is less costly than basic sanitation and, therefore, more popular in some quarters? To top it all, the latest regarding irradiation is the investigation of some postal workers who allegedly suffered serious health problems. The suspected culprit was allegedly irradiation. These postal employees worked in post offices that irradiated all the mail they processed following the terrorist Anthrax attacks. There were no reports, though, that these employees were munching envelopes during lunch.

Passengers, on board several cruise ships, have repeatedly experienced gastrointestinal virus outbreaks of almost epidemic proportions. Will the FDA recommend anytime soon that cruise ships and passengers and crews be irradiated prior to each sailing? The "lucky" sailors on the HMS Bounty only had to worry about scurvy, which they took care of by spiking their rum with lime juice. Had they instead been confronted with irradiation, they might possibly have mutinied sooner. A national daily publication recently reported that the food industry is lobbying the FDA to change the wording on the labels of irradiated foods. It seems they would like to replace the word "irradiated" with "electronically pasteurized." Could this be because it might sound like a "newer, improved" version of Louis Pasteur' rabies vaccine? What would be the benefit of calling, for example, a bank robbery an "unauthorized cash withdrawal?" Unless it gave the perpetrators what Rodney Dangerfield craved—Respect.

The endless and continuous stream of news highlighting more and more myriad recommendations brings to light newer controversies, newer reports of past, present, and future side effects, after effects, countermeasures, counter countermeasures, and retractions, etc.

If one chooses to apply the myriad recommendations, advice, etc., in order to "keep healthy," one may eventually have need of the Pentagon mainframe to keep track of everything that would be needed to be done 24-7, with no time left to even go to the bathroom. All of this effort may still be an exercise in futility, as it would maintain the myth of One-Size-Fits-All, as well as pursuing the Chimaera of the Symptom Suppression Jihad.

Once again, could it be that in spite of good intentions, and all the scientific progress, we may still not have even a glimpse of the Big Picture of the consequences of the Big Bang, i.e., the inconceivably unlimited concept of the Universe and all of its laws and interconnections? Yet, Kant thought that we humans are indeed bound by some limitations. Should this be, indeed, the case, then it may be preferable to seek mutual assistance by supporting and co-operating with the "limited picture" we have in view, rather than trying to duplicate it, second guess it, and even attempt to counteract it. Let alone that we still have no clue of the Big Picture. After all the Big Banger of the Universe is still unidentified, at least scientifically. Futile second-guessing, counteracting, etc., may be creating, after all, more problems than providing solutions.

It may not just be a case of deliberately ignoring the Universal Law of "Cause and Effect," but that we simply seem to have limited knowledge of both causes and effects. But this seemingly insufficient knowledge does not seem to discourage some from "causing" knowingly or not, and as to the effects, they might as well repeat after Doris Day *"Que Sera, Sera."*

Could it be that Voltaire, the eighteenth century French philosopher and writer, had also some doubts about the extent of our collective knowledge when he said, *"Doctors are men who prescribe medicines of which they know little, to cure diseases of which they know less, in human beings of whom they know nothing."* One may wonder if it is our collective knowledge that is incomplete or if the health givers just gave up on counting on the health recipients to quit overwhelming their mind body system. Maybe, and probably, both.

Some may ask, if a human being is such a marvellous and perfect creation, and potentially indestructible since it is self-sustaining, self-maintaining, self-repairing and self-regenerating, how come, at times, it can get so screwed up? This happens most likely through the inherent Free Will/Power of Choice. Some may indeed choose to overwhelm all these attributes and manage to screw things up. Dr. Weil pretty well said that our body will serve us well unless it is overwhelmed, mainly by us.

This wonderful creation has built in all kinds of "warning lights and buzzers", i.e., it emits myriad of warning signals about anything and everything that attempts to overwhelm it, as well as encouraging signals about everything that supports it. Some choose to ignore and even suppress the first, while choosing to remain unaware of the second. Ignoring or suppressing these signals is figuratively tantamount to masking you car's gauges and warning lights with duct tape and/or pulling electrical wires, or worse, reaching for ear plugs when the home smoke detector goes off. The third category of signals is that of gratification and joy when everything is functioning harmoniously.

All these signals are basically transmitted through:

- Body senses

- Bodily functions

- Intuition/Feelings.

These signals are emitted non-stop 24-7 from womb to grave. One may perceive the signals being transmitted when one chooses to have body, mind, and intuition/feelings aligned on the same "wave length," and "talking to each other and, thus, having their act together." Only then, may one choose to receive these signals, and after a holistic self-observation, and having applied some deduction and common sense, finally interpret them. Then vet, coordinate, process, and finally respond to them, through one's Free Will/Power of Choice.

When interpreting and vetting these signals it is vital to separate the wheat from the chaff once more, i.e., separate our very own knowledge, thoughts, and experiences, from other people's information, opinions, dogmas, habits, etc., some of which we might have already adopted as our own. Simply put, it would be similar to eliminating the static that may pollute our internal communications channels. Maybe the advice of the first century AD celebrated Roman satirist Persius applies here: *"Nor Ask Any Opinion But Your Own" (Nec te quaesiveris extra)*.

An additional benefit, of receiving and processing the transmitted signals, is that it enables you to have an informed, intelligent and effective dialogue with your physician or health caregiver. You are, therefore, able to help your physician help you, and nobody can do it better than you, just as suggested by the Babylonian tablets.

All this may seem to some as a complex and even impossible task, actually it may prove to be very simple and even automatic, and eventually may be carried out spontaneously and instantly, without even giving it a thought if we so choose.

Each one of us is the sole architect of our health or lack thereof, just as "designed." All things being equal, and if each one of us functioned perfectly according to our "design specs," then possibly one would not then need more health care than Adam and Eve allegedly needed in the Garden of Eden, before their lease was abruptly cancelled. Furthermore, there is no mention in Genesis about HMOs, Medicare, and Medicaid, availability in the Garden of Eden. In case anybody asks, apparently there was no Hillary Care either

The TROIKA of body, mind, and intuition/feelings,

that can achieve the above, if it so chooses, may be compared to a philharmonic. The body represents the instruments/band, the mind represents the conductor whose baton is Free/Will/Power of Choice, the intuition/feelings represents the composer, and the resulting love and joy of creating melody is represented by the applause, i.e., being and feeling great. When all three perform in concert (no pun intended) a perfect harmonious melody always results. Each one of us is a one of a kind philharmonic and its performance relies entirely on our Free Will/Power of Choice. Some may be reminded, while appreciating the wonders of this Philharmonic, by these words of good old Billy the Bard: *"THERE ARE MORE THINGS IN HEAVEN AND EARTH HORATIO, THAN ARE DREAMT OF IN YOUR PHILOSOPHY."*

There was a teenager who was an avid car enthusiast and deeply in love with his dad's fast sport sedan and the unlimited privileges of access that went with it. This teenager would frequently get up at 3:00 a.m. (for many teenagers that may be a heavy duty sacrifice) when the city was free of any noise pollution, to listen with loving care to the car's idling engine for the slightest unorthodox noise due to timing, carburettor, tappets, etc. Then, he would drive it through the deserted streets, trying to detect chassis, suspension, tire, or any other unorthodox, noises. Then came the sudden bursts of maximum acceleration to ensure there was not the slightest hesitation, let alone stalling. Then steering, brakes, etc., were checked. When it came to the maintenance manual's recommendations, this kid was more Catholic than the Pope. Nothing but top grade, fuel, lubricants, fluids, spark plugs tires, etc., and the icing on the cake was an immaculate wax and polish. The rewards, though, were incomparable performance at all times, total reliability, and looks of jealous admiration, from all quarters, culminating in endless fun and pure joy.

The kid was simply very much in love with it and very protective. Not to mention that the kid was also a formidable, and accident free, street dragger. Can one afford to be less protective of one's own body and love it less, and most importantly miss out on all the fun and Joy? That is, HEALTH.

Similarly, an avid skier might feel this way about his skis, and lovingly always check the bottoms of his skis for any gouges and fill them in, use the best and most appropriate wax, sharpen the edges with the best diamond sharpener, ensure one hundred percent function of the bindings, etc. Then, on the slope he becomes one with the ski; feels everything the ski "feels"; and knows that no one else comes close to knowing what is best for his skis and the ecstasy he derives from them. Here again the outcome can be endless fun and pure joy. Those, who love to hunt or fish, most likely act the same way with their guns or fishing gear, and with the same results. The same goes for cyclists and their bikes, skate boarders and their skate boards, golfers and their clubs, etc., etc.

It may seem quite obvious that the common denominator of the above motivations, and the resulting fun and joy, is loving and enjoying what one is doing, as well as loving what one is doing it with. Primarily this includes

LIVING, i.e., LIVING IN HEALTH, WITH A SOUND BODY AND MIND.

Just imagine that skis are symbolizing the skier's physical and mental health, and then try to picture the skier's delirious ecstasy, while schussing all out down a Utah slope in chest-deep, super-light powder. WOW! All those multiple orgasms.

Common sense might indicate that in devoting more, not less, loving care to our physical and mental health, we stand to reap more, not less, endless fun and pure joy, consistently and uninterruptedly.

The question is, can one really afford to do more for skiing and skis than for living with a healthy body and mind? And the answer is, as always: "It Is Simply a Matter of Choice." Your Choice.

Stress

Stress may be the most insidiously influential of the Six Key Factors affecting human health, and can be powerfully devastating while greatly affecting the other five factors.

There are basically two sources of stress. One is Self-Contradiction and the resulting Internal Conflict, and the other is Fear, which is the supreme terrorist of all time. They both have numerous derivatives and guises. They are mostly consequences of one's omnipresent and absolute Free Will/Power of Choice (i.e., one's own choices), and therefore self created. As Mr. Spock might say to Captain Kirk, "Captain, if one can choose to create stress, it is logical that one can choose to prevent or eliminate it." "Stress Management" is but part and parcel of the Symptom Suppression Jihad, i.e., an aspirin for acute appendicitis. To some, managing stress is not unlike trying to manage a fire in your house, instead of putting it out or preventing it in the first place.

It is being repeatedly reported that obesity, having reached epidemic proportions, continues to spread and with it, its most direct consequences such as diabetes, cancer, and cardiovascular diseases, just to name a few. Science seems to attribute it mainly to eating and drinking excesses, both in quantity and quality, as well as insufficient physical activity.

According to JAMA because of inadequate diet and physical activity, obesity caused over 400,000 preventable (a matter of choice...again) deaths a year, while smoking caused 460,000 preventable deaths, and the difference is that smoking is declining, while obesity is on the rise, and both are preventable.

There are those who think that obesity may be initiated by one's state of mind, i.e., frustration, stress, etc., which in turn may affect eating, drinking, and lifestyle. There are some who after a somewhat protracted period of unhappiness, anguish, and frustration, in one word stress, may notice that their clothes get tighter and tighter, a potential precursor that their perceptible weight gain might snowball into an avalanche, i.e., OBESITY.

Many may be familiar with the renowned French

delicacy *"pâte de foie gras,"* which literally means "Fat Liver Pate," and is indeed extra fatty, processed, Goose liver. The geese destined to produce it are deliberately stressed, practically tortured, and are immobilized in tight quarters, and endlessly fed, until they balloon and their liver is so diseased with the excess fat that it can no longer process, hence fat liver.

It would appear that, maybe, stress works on the Geese as well, since it does not spare them from either obesity or disease.

Medical science keeps on reporting more and more about the ravages of stress on our physical and mental health all the way to depression and worse. It has also been reported that this struggling and straining also seriously undermines and compromises our autoimmune system. That is tantamount to undermining simultaneously the military, the police, homeland security, and the laws of our nation. It does not take a lot of imagination to picture the terrifying outcome of such a scenario. After all, it would seem, according to the available scientific information, that most diseases are triggered because somewhere, somehow, the autoimmune system has been compromised/overwhelmed and failed to do its job. It is probably not too difficult for many, if not most to guess, who causes most, if not all, of the compromising and overwhelming. However, for those who might find guessing a challenge, they may want to look into the closest mirror and utter the classic,

"We have seen the enemy, and the enemy is us."

Fear, one of the two main sources of stress, may well

be considered self-created since it is mostly contingent on our Free Will/Power of Choice (thoughts, words, deeds). It is also, often, a direct derivative of our self-contradictions and the consequent internal conflict.

However, some seem to have, an overwhelming at times, fear of death, and this fear may be allowed to become a source of great stress. That too is a matter of choice. Those who fear death may consider some possibly prevalent and even acceptable points of view that may prove helpful in assisting them in choosing not to fear death.

Those who may be fans of the Ninth Circuit Court, i.e., that is members of the Zeus Club, may find some solace in science and its findings. Interpreting cosmologists' assertions, one could sum it up as that since Infinite Energy In Perpetual Motion is underlying everything in the Universe, while it keeps it together, there is no ingress or egress (not even a fire exit), i.e., no loss (let alone extinction) of this Energy in the Universe, just its perpetual motion change and expansion. Accordingly, therefore, nothing stops or disappears or, if you will dies. There is just motion, change, and transformation. Everything changes in the Universe, all the time, except for change itself. Some in the recycling industry, might view the Universe as the ultimate infinite jumbo recycling plant. Technically, therefore, there is no death, or if you will, no disappearance, activity cessation, or energy loss, just change and transformation. However, since scientists have not as yet identified let alone questioned the Big Banger, they are unable to tell us what we might be transformed or changed into. But those with an insatiable curiosity can always, in the meantime, consult Shirley McLaine, or even Pythagoras should he show up.

Those who may not be members of the Zeus Club, may do well to remember, that prior to his abrupt departure, the Nazarene Master guaranteed his fans reservations at his paternal estates' many resort mansions. However, there was no mention of air mile credits as well, not even for frequent fliers like Shirley McLaine.

There are, also, those whose views may belong somewhere in-between the previous two groups. But all may, if they so choose, call their particular choice, religion. Yet there may be those who may feel most reassured just by this simple ancient Tibetan monk saying:

"Show me a man who is not afraid to die, and I will show you a religious man."

For some, stress may be rendered irrelevant by simply being in charge at all times of their Free Will/Power of Choice, while keeping in mind that everything they think, say, and do has natural (Universal Law of Cause and Effect) consequences. The resulting responsibility may in turn provide unrestricted liberty without self-contradictions, internal conflicts, and the resulting fear, not to mention the "fashionable if not popular" depressions.

Speaking of depressions, a national daily publication reported that in Europe and France, in particular, they are concerned with the ever-expanding use of tranquilizers and antidepressants. According to the International Narcotics Control Board, an agency financed by the United Nations, Western Europe is practically the biggest consumer of tranquilizers and antidepressants on the planet, with France leading the charge. (Could it be that they are not consuming enough "freedom fries"?).

According to IMS Health, a health care data and consulting outfit, pill-for-pill Americans consume eighteen percent fewer pills than the French but spend over three hundred percent as much. As per a French government estimate, tranquilizers and antidepressants cost their national medical insurance system $20.9 BILLION a year, while it had a $17.7 BILLION deficit.

French, and other Europeans, are attempting to slow down this cataclysm through regulation, and publicity campaigns to persuade consumers and health givers to cut down a bit on the pills.

Meanwhile, back at the ranch in the good old USA, "only" forty-eight (for now) of available tranquilizers and antidepressants pills are prescribed also to children, talking about "the sins of the fathers visiting the sons." Some may view all of this, as but a dangerous and harmful exercise in futility, in full compliance with the Symptom Suppression Jihad without exterminating the main underlying cause, STRESS.

More recently, the FDA issued warnings about ten (for starters) major antidepressant drugs whose possible risks include increased suicidal tendencies. These drugs are prescribed to both children and adults. Some may wonder whether Bin Laden's second in command the "good" Dr. Zawahri, is importing these drugs, and feeding them to the Al Qaeda and Hamas suicide bombers.

Dr. Bruce McEwen director of the neuroendocrinology laboratory of the Rockefeller University in Manhattan, and author of a new book, *The End of Stress As We Know It*, has said that prolonged or severe stress has been shown to weaken the immune system, strain the heart, damage memory cells in the brain, and deposit fat at the waist (a risk factor for heart disease, cancer, and other illnesses) rather than the hips and buttocks. Stress has been implicated in ageing, depression, heart disease, rheumatoid arthritis, and diabetes, among other illnesses.

According to Dr. McEwen the best ways to cope, turns out to be the time honoured ones—eat sensibly, get plenty of sleep, exercise regularly, stop at one martini, and stay away from cigarettes. He concluded,

"It's a matter of making choices in your life."

One could possibly summarize Dr. McEwen's findings on stress quite laconically as follows:

1   Healthy mind in a healthy body.

2   *"All Measure Excels"* (Aristotle's "golden" equilibrium between excesses)

3   You get to choose.

Some may, therefore, conclude that Being In Charge Of Yourself, may come in real handy each time you get to choose to render stress irrelevant.

The other five factors affecting human health consist of:

- Everything ingested

- Everything breathed

- Physical activity

- State of mind

- Lifestyle

The "Philharmonic" may be gainfully enlisted to provide health through the following three steps:

1 Reactivating clear and direct communications with one's "Philharmonic", i.e., starting by accepting and receiving its signals and verifying their origin, interpreting them, then investigating them with common sense, and then responding, and finally looking for feedback. Eventually these communications will get clearer and stronger (practice makes perfect) and function as automatically as blinking. The confirmation of full, clear, and direct communication, with the Philharmonic, is the loving and enjoying every minute of it, knowing full well it will never give you a bum steer.

2 Top priority in communicating may be the choice to neither ignore or suppress the signals and the symptoms you experience, i.e., "remove the duct

tape covering the engine trouble lights, and reconnect the buzzer wires" as well as choosing to refrain from: "This thing bugs me and quickly give me a pill to make it disappear now, and don't bother me with the details and/or consequences." The findings of recent medical research indicated that eczema symptoms may be caused by a deficiency in the body's natural and automatic production of antibiotics. If these findings are taken at face value, one might ask, "Is this a loud and clear enough communication from the body that something is not clicking, or what?" Yet some will just take pills and apply ointments on the lesions in order to suppress the symptoms, and that may even produce additional and possibly different symptoms, i.e., collateral damage/side effects and thus propagate further a vicious circle, and maybe chronically so. In short, the "band-aid/pills" to suppress the symptoms may prove to be but a Trojan Horse.

3   When communicating, it is vital to choose our own thoughts and experiences over those of others, which we may or not have already unwittingly claimed as our very own. At times, some "outside" thoughts, views, and ideas, may be chosen once "vetted by the Philharmonic."

Picture a healthy, fit person, who is athletically inclined, and who loves long distance running. Then imagine this person agreeing to put casts on both legs, hip to toes for a year, and with the use of crutches the feet will never touch the ground. After twelve months, the casts are removed and the person is invited to participate in the Boston Marathon the next morning. Yeah right! The old USE IT OR LOOSE IT concept, alas, is omnipresent and always valid. Eventually, if and when that person chooses to run marathons after rehabilitation, physiotherapy, and training, may do so successfully.

This legs in casts parable may apply to some who have been ignoring and suppressing the signals and symptoms provided automatically by their Philharmonic, i.e., they did not use it and so lost it, meaning communication. With practice though, if so chosen, full communication with your Philharmonic can be gradually restored. It is often claimed that practice makes perfect, and in this case everything then, will eventually be on "automatic pilot."

The lack of adequate internal communication may cause fear to some about their health, feeling they have no control over it. As a result, they might be more susceptible to third party information and experiences, dogmas, and generally embracing the One-Size-Fits-All myth. Since they have no "internal communication" that would either confirm or dissolve their fear, they may tend to follow as many third party recommendations as possible and subject themselves to myriad tests, and agonize while awaiting the results. Such a situation may contribute little to eliminating stress, not to mention thinking all the time about the realization of their worst fears. Many such unwelcome scenarios, may have been prevented if signals had been received from the Philharmonic's DEW (Distant Early Warning) Line. The DEW LINE never fails to warn, (unless its communications are not received or ignored) and, therefore, there should not be any "Pearl Harbour" health scenarios, i.e., sudden catastrophic illnesses.

- Medical science over time has interpreted or speculated about some common body messages, such as the cravings of a pregnant woman. The speculation is that the body goes on "overdrive" to protect mother and baby by amplifying manifestations of its current related needs. The craving being possibly just one expression or signal of these needs.

- Pregnancy provides probably some of the simpler illustrations of body signals. Medical science has speculated that the "morning sickness" may be a similar situation where the body, in a protective mode, is trying to indicate that at this time, nothing, or something in particular, should or should not be ingested.

- Medical science has also speculated that prehistoric women were blessed with easy, simple, and painless birthing. This was allegedly attributed to lifestyle and physical activity.

- Some people responded to the first by abusing or trivializing or even ridiculing these "frivolous cravings," which have also been blamed for prenatal overweight.

- Some people responded to the second with Thalidomide.

- Some people responded to the third with

prenatal physical exercises and weight control diets.

Possibly for some others, the body messages were not quite received, or decoded or adequately responded to.

Everything ingested

Once communications have been established and the "Philharmonic" is fully operational, some may eventually and gradually experience the following as it pertains to food and drink, and everything else ingested for that matter:

1   An automatic or instinctive adherence to a single diet practically consisting solely of eating and drinking everything you love and enjoy, as much as you like, whenever and wherever you feel like it and at the same time rejecting everything you do not like at all times. Gradually and "wondrously" anything "harmful" will find itself on the list of everything you do not like. At the same time, the "acquired palate" syndrome (which is born of and/ or conducive to habit forming excesses) as well as the addictive pursuit of a taste buds "buzz" would be rendered irrelevant. Such a diet, constantly and automatically, will be changing according to your changes and those of your needs without you giving it a second thought. If this sounds incredible to some, then our miraculous sympathetic nervous system, which is witnessed and experienced by all non-stop throughout our lives, and which is a full

member of the "Philharmonic" may as well sound equally incredible.

This sort of diet will also keep Aristotle smiling, as it may enhance your health by inherently encouraging variety, thus automatically providing a safeguard against excesses, just like Saddam Hussein's sleeping "diet," which protected him. Allegedly, every night he slept in a different place to avoid receiving an offer he could not refuse from his "fan club." He got "nailed" when he restricted his sleeping diet to a spider hole or two.

Additionally, some may have experienced and/or observed that human beings intrinsically pursue hedonism. Hedonism may be manifested in everything and anywhere, unless suppressed or bypassed by our Free Will/Power of Choice. For some hedonism may prove capital whenever they eat and drink. Some may have, occasionally, observed that whenever they are eating something with genuine (supported by your instincts/feelings) great gusto, and are over salivating and crying WOW...YUMMY, after each mouthful, they may have probably experienced the following automatically:

- No gulping down food fast.

- No overeating.

- Not necessary to spell relief, R...O...L...A...I...D...S, or otherwise.

- A feeling of full restoration and energy surplus.

- A hedonistic feeling of well being.

Similarly some may, after an hour or two of a highly enjoyable fast game of squash, gulp down two or three beers with the same above mentioned gusto, and with a similar consequential experience.

Others, on the other hand while watching a ball game on TV, may be mechanically taking small sips of beer for hours, not only they might not feel any hedonism, but on the contrary they may even feel drowsy, etc.

Hedonism can, at times, be experienced when gulping just plain iced water on a hot day.

Hedonism is equally gratifying in physical activities, sports, and for that matter, in everything else one is engaged in. Some may conclude that hedonism is the stamp of approval of the "Philharmonic."

2   Consequently there may be no need to own a scale or loosen and/or upsize your entire wardrobe. The "Philharmonic" will add to your comfort and pleasure by automatically providing you with the optimal weight exclusively for YOU as well as maintaining it. Good-bye and good riddance calorie, carbohydrate, fat, and artificial sweetener (just to name a few) Gestapo.

3   There will probably be no urgency any more to compulsively channel surf for the commercials about the latest pills against heartburn, constipation, diarrhoea, etc., or for supplements, herbs, diets, etc. Some may discover and conclude that all the diet gurus in the universe don't come even close

(light years away) to YOUR "Philharmonic" in providing YOU the diet that will benefit YOU alone the most. Some may speculate that this is pure fantasy or plain wishful thinking. They might want to consider our sympathetic nervous system. Incessantly and automatically, it executes myriad miraculous functions for the optimum benefit of our mind body team, pro-actively, actively, and reactively, and even at times in spite of us. On the other hand, our Philharmonic, when in "concert," performs interactively, as we choose with equally wondrous results for our optimum benefit.

4   With the "Philharmonic" in concert, eventually all food and drink purveyors, drug manufacturers, will be but your "subcontractors," if and when you say so, and you will be telling them "which cow ate the cabbage" not the other way around, no matter the labels, the ads, the commercials, and whatever a "Baghdad Bob" may recommend. Eventually the people as always will prevail and again validate Abe's *"You Cannot Fool All the People All the Time."* Henry Ford had said that people could choose any color they wanted for their Model T, provided it was black. Later through the Seventies and on, Detroit seemingly suffered from the "*Father Knows Best* Syndrome," i.e., "We know what is the best car for you, we built it, and you will just have to buy it." Then along came the Japanese, who basically said to the people, "Tell us what kind of a car do you fancy, and we will build it for you." Most are familiar with the aftermath. Detroit today is scrambling to catch up. Some may believe that

it is only a matter of time when many may choose to no longer place themselves, at the mercy of the proverbial " thirty second TV commercials," and reverse the tables and start dictating to the suppliers by precisely Choosing For Themselves what is it exactly that they want. In order to make it happen some may call on their innate gift of discrimination amplified by experience and enhanced by common sense. This may help discern the following in all information sources i.e.. communications, promotions, and advertising in general:

- Overtones of Goebbels and Pavlovian techniques no matter how subtle

- Promotion of the Lemming Syndrome

- Promotion and encouragement of dependency, as amply demonstrated in the Tobacco class actions

It is self-evident that it is the only way one can make it happen. On the other hand, as easily observed, this may not be happening now or anytime soon through regulations, legislation, class action, or any other lawsuits alone, since they just provide additional expense, aggravation, and suffering endlessly. Ask Sisyphus, because he tried something like that, he is still at it, and will continue FOREVER.

There are probably some, who might appreciate a vivid illustration, and even a confirmation of the above. They may find it in the popular movie *"Super Size Me,"* which was launched nation wide in the spring of 2004. In this entertaining and factual documentary movie, the central character volunteered to deliberately alter his dietary habits for thirty days and mimic the prevalent, and seemingly, permanent eating habits and fads of a vast majority of the population. Fortunately, for the volunteer, the thirty-day trial was conducted under clinical guidance and supervision. These eating fads had already sparked a lot of controversy and finger pointing in many quarters. They allegedly contribute significantly to obesity, which has reached epidemic proportions, and is still rising. In addition to obesity, with all its ramifications, they also contributed to severe and even chronic ill health in various forms as well as dependency and addiction, all of which are rampant nationwide. This real reality movie seems to reconfirm and make the following points crystal clear:

- Excess harms.

- Lack of variety is very risky and can also be harmful.

- Both excess and lack of variety can lead to obesity.

- Both excess and lack of variety can lead to holistic health deterioration.

- Both excess and lack of variety can lead to addiction.

- Diet and addiction, like everything else, are always a matter of one's choice.

- The mind and body team, indeed, signalled

repeatedly, and in many ways, their disapproval of the volunteer's new habits. Initially, through feelings of malaise, here and there and then followed with protestations and demonstrations by the senses and the bodily functions

- The volunteer kept (for the sake of the experiment) ignoring the signals. As a result, actual physical and mental health impairments began to appear. Clinical tests by a team of three doctors and a dietician confirmed these impairments and uncovered even more. One impairment, however, was also confirmed by someone not belonging to the medical profession; his girlfriend who seemed to suggest that he either get off his thirty day diet or he get on Viagra.

Who knows, maybe the Viagra folks might even encourage and sponsor the volunteer to promote for them in a sequel movie, "Super Size Me II" or "Super Size Me, Too."

While we are on the subject, Slick Willy, during his many media interviews about his new book, kept repeating that the most inexcusable aspect of his regrettable (so he said) affair with Monica was that he did it simply, because "he could do it." Most likely there would have been no stained blue dress, "it depends what is IS," or impeachment, had he followed a diet like in the movie simply because then, "he could not have done it."

- One can choose to overwhelm one's mind and body team, or support it. As always, it is simply a matter of one's choice.

- Due to the fact that this was an experiment conducted in a clinical environment, and that there were constant discussions and information exchanged between the health givers and the volunteer, the wonderful outcome in restoring his health is self-evident.

- In real life, those indulging in dietary excesses, etc., are not conducting clinical experiments. They just end up asking the doctor to relieve their symptoms of discomfort with the proverbial "magic pill," and no questions asked, followed by the inevitable combined domino and ripple effects of deteriorating health. All taken for granted as part of *"c'est la vie."*

- All this seems to confirm, once more, the wisdom of the ancient Babylonian tablet, which indicates that the best physician is the one who talks the most with his patient.

There are some, who through denial of their Free Will/ Power of Choice, may ignore the body's or, rather, the "Philharmonic's" signals by claiming the "no (not my) fault syndrome clause." Some may claim it is because of what has been inherited, or because of some addiction, or their genes, or old age, or their environment, etc. A recent book on obesity states that if someone is obese it is not their fault, it is that of their genes and that of the cultural influences one is exposed to. This thesis could be a bonanza for the tort warriors of the obese people suing fast food chains for starters. These lawsuits claim that the fast food chains, knowingly and deliberately, fed the claimants excessively fatty, addictive foods that led to their obesity. By now, the tort warriors can also probably launch a civil rights lawsuit for discrimination against their clients' genes and violation of their culture. So much for the Free Will/Power of Choice, as well as for the Law of Cause and Effect. However, for those who choose to deny the Free Will/Power of Choice, this "not my fault" approach could be a powerful "opiate" for the obese.

The "genes effect" after attempting to justify obesity, is now coming to the rescue of cheating spouses. A more recent scientific "finding" seems to blame one's genes for conjugal infidelity. Some compulsive cheating spouses might welcome this finding as a sort of a Vioxx pill against the good old "Mea Culpa" condition as well as responsibility in general. It might also cut down on the amounts of divorce settlements and divorce lawyer fees. In both cases i.e., obesity and infidelity it might seem to some that it is just another futile attempt to transfer the inherent and absolute Free Will/Power of Choice of human beings to some gene here and there, even when a gene attempts to merely hint at times at some predisposition. There goes Billy again,

" *To Be Or Not To Be*," and that **is** the **Choice**.

Dr. David L. Katz, a professor at the Yale School of Medicine, and author of *"The Way To Eat"*, *who also* recently wrote *Advances in Pharmacotherapy*, *writes that even the revolution of Genomic Medicine, will never prove, ultimately, effective in the control of epidemic obesity. Only environmental and behavioural changes will take us where we need to go. "* Dr. Katz's statement will probably get some flak from the "Flat Earth Society," as well from those engaged in class actions against restaurant chains. On the other hand, his statement may be translated and summarized by some as follows:

- Remember who you are.

- Review your original design (as created by the Big Bang itself) "specs and maintenance manual."

- Tune in to your "Philharmonic" and choose (feel free to use your Free Will/Power of Choice of choice).

- Forget the rest.

Many may wonder at the ceaseless and futile efforts of those with obesity problems to locate the miracle pill or silver bullet every where and anywhere except within themselves and their free will/power of choice. Maybe that all time paragon of orators, good old Demosthenes the Athenian who gave Philip the Deuce of Macedonia and his son Al the Great such a hard time, has the answer. He stated

"Nothing is easier than self-deceit".

Just as a reminder, Demosthenes the great orator was also the fellow with a severe "lingual" dysfunction, he stuttered like hell, but apparently he rejected treatments with hormones, steroids, or "lingual" Viagra (maybe he was wary of side and after effects). Instead he opted for speech therapy by swirling beach pebbles in his mouth while talking to himself during long strolls on deserted beaches. If only he could show up to deliver a virulent Philippic oration at the next national silver bullet and magic pill convention. In the event Demosthenes can not make it due to prior commitments, maybe Arkansas Governer Mike Huckabee could be invited to step in.

Early in 2005 Governor Huckabee was interviewed on a major network about his triumph over obesity and the weight loss of 110lbs, Competing in marathons and also his new book on his experience. Apparently it took his physician's ultimatum that if he did not change lifestyle and conquer his obesity, in 10 years he would trade his Governor's mansion for one much smaller **six feet under.**

To some, possibly Mike Huckabee's most significant statement was that he conquered by TAKING CHARGE. This entailed selective nutrition devoid of excesses appropriate physical activities, as well as adopting an equally appropriate integrated lifestyle.

He emphasized that he did not accomplish this through futile dieting. Apparently through effort and deliberate consistent, structured tactics, he achieved victory and now enjoys, vitality and a joyous wellbeing, Some may conclude that had his own "Philharmonic" been in full concert earlier on, possibly his experience could have been innately more effortless and possibly more joyous i.e., on automatic pilot. Now that the Governor has written a book, it maybe time that he stars in a documentary entitled " Downsize Me!", which could possibly get nominated for an Oscar (as did the "Super size Me ' documentary movie), and actually win. Some may conclude that the Governor hit the jackpot of his life by choosing to TAKE CHARGE of himself and his health.

The efforts of the fans of gastrointestinal surgery and/or massive abdominal liposuction (with all their ramifications), the silver bullet hunters, and the blame-and-sue-everything-and-anything artists, may remind of the fifth century BC Persian king Xerxes' exercise in futility.

Xerxes, having brutally suppressed rebellions in Egypt and Babylon, decided to add to his vast and powerful empire the Greek States. To this end, he marched his armies (well over a million troops) to the edge of Asia Minor, where the Persian navy would transport them over to the European side and then march all the way to Athens. However, a heavy and prolonged sea storm caused his army and navy delays and damages, which infuriated the mighty and proud king who decided to teach the sea a lesson so that it would quit agitating. He ordered that the sea be given a myriad of lashings. The whipping, though, did not exactly stop the storm in its tracks as he expected. Eventually, much later, the storm died down and Xerxes proceeded all the way to Athens, where ironically, he got clobbered by the Athenian navy, and then made a one eighty and headed home. One might say that this was the Ancient Greek "Battle of the Midway." For those, to whom the Xerxes story sounds all Greek, quoting Sir Winston Churchill may illustrate the frustrating futility of supporting the Flat Earth Society, when it opposes Dr. Katz's views.

Sir Winston Churchill was Chancellor of the Exchequer (something like our Secretary of the Treasury) in the 1920s, and he was advocating cutting taxes across the board and in a speech to Parliament he said, *"We contend, that for a nation to try to tax itself into prosperity is like a man standing in a bucket and trying to lift himself up by the handles."* Had our Treasury Secretary emeritus Paul O'Neil been around at the time, he might have written a book about Winnie as the blind hero among the deaf. In Churchillian terms, the first step in fighting obesity might be "drop the handles and get the hell out of the bucket."

It is amazing, or maybe not, how everybody seems to conspire to cater to those who might not want to get the hell out of the bucket. According to scientists, recent animal studies show that using artificial sweeteners may throw off people's inherent ability to monitor how many calories they consume. A recent Purdue University study confirms the above, and also raises concerns that a similar phenomenon may occur with processed foods featuring reduced fats and/or carbohydrates. Again, one may conclude that trying to counter and/or fool the mind-body system is at best counterproductive. The "Philharmonic" simply cannot be outperformed when it is in concert. After all, it belongs to UBB's Gizmo of Ultimate Perfection a.k.a. GUP.

Some may feel like paraphrasing JFK for all those seeking obesity's silver bullet, "Ask not what others and things can do for your health and your obesity, ask what you can do for your health and your obesity." Surprise, surprise, a recent study in Ohio indicated that extremely obese youngsters can have heart abnormalities that put them at serious risk of heart attacks. Although many may not be surprised, they might ask the same question congressmen often ask on the hill,

"Where Is the Outrage?"

In 2001, Stanford University researchers confirmed that food ads on TV (let alone other media) can influence the food choices of preschool kids. The question this research poses is how much do these ads contribute to child and youth obesity or at the very least its predisposition? It would seem that Marion Nestle, Professor of Nutrition at New York University, agrees wholeheartedly with the Stanford findings. On account of this point of view, it is safe to speculate that the professor is in no way connected with the Nestle food Titan and major advertiser.

The CDC is also engaged in the debate by sponsoring a major study of the effects of advertising on the diets and health of children that could possibly lead to government oversight of such advertising.

The World Health Organisation which joined the above via its 2003 report on nutrition and chronic diseases prevention also confirmed the link between junk food marketing and childhood obesity. The WHO went on to recommend government action.

More recently the European Union (including Rummie's "Old Europe") also joined the above "Coalition of the Willing" as it is considering to impose restrictions on marketing to children unless the industry does it first.

Could it be that Dr. Goebbels is still around?

On the other hand, some may realise that as businesses go, the food manufacturers and their advertisers have one thing in common. No where in their mission statements does it seem to state that they are committed to fight obesity, ill health, chronic diseases and addiction. It merely emphasizes their very *raison d'être* – to make money - and therefore act accordingly.

The current widespread obesity and ill health avalanche seems to have prompted governments and institutions to take leave of their lethargy by attempting to mediate the conflict between business and consumers i.e. in favor of public interest.

Some, however, feel that it could possibly culminate into just another snail-paced exercise in futility, and too little too late at that. Possibly the only way to tackle this Gordian knot, the required Sword of Alexander, would be the for the people (and in this case, the parents in particular) to Be In Charge of Themselves and dictate to Business in Billy the Bard's own words "To Be or Not To Be" and conclude with what Klink and Schultz might have said "DS (short for Dat Sit), Zee Felfet Gloves Are Off, No Morrr Misterr Nice Guy."

As already mentioned, common sense and the vetting process are the key components of the "Philharmonic's" orchestration. This would include being inquisitive about what is ingested, reading carefully labels for ingredients, additives, processes, etc. It would also include noticing, evaluating, and noting, all the feedback that the body is providing. However, one may find choosing a difficult task due to the inexhaustible plethora of the so-called new and improved items, followed faithfully by the inevitable findings of side effects and after effects, or at best "inaccurate" claims. It is no longer simple to select the most beneficial or least harmful items. Track record longevity is one basic initial indicator, e.g., for thousands of years olive oil has been consumed with relish and safety and even alleged health benefits.

On the other hand, imagine a chemist coming up with a new, improved, and "tastier" salad/cooking oil (let alone dressing) "that is really good for you, which also prevents Attention Deficit Syndrome." Later, research shows that this salad oil causes schizophrenia, then, still later, somebody else provides a "tasty" synthetic salad vinegar to cancel out the schizophrenia factor, but which later produced its own manic depression symptoms, and on and on. You get the picture.

Plain common sense may indicate that olive oil may be a safer and possibly tastier bet. Through the millennia, it appears there were no claims that it caused everything from gonorrhoea to epilepsy, to depression, or anything else for that matter. At the same time, it may be helpful to remember that nothing is safe in excess. If this very hypothetical salad oil "parable" might seem far fetched and/or ridiculous, a daily glance at the news media may very well render it both realistic and even routine. Equally observable is that such a scenario may very well apply to medication as well.

Following a several years long study, the European Union concluded that the well over fifty percent, reduction of stomach cancer incidence was mainly due to improved dietary habits, and improved oversight of food sources, processes, labels, etc.

A similar common sense approach may apply to medication as well. Aspirin has been around for over a hundred years and is still popular, considered beneficial, and relatively harmless, unless consumed excessively. It is based on an extract from the willow tree bark. Hippocratic medicine in ancient Greece widely used this extract for its analgesic and other benefits. Also for thousands of years, the inhabitants of the South American rain forests used the bark of the Cinchona tree for its medicinal benefits. Its extract, Quinine, was modern medicine's prime weapon against Malaria during most of the twentieth century.

One could say that both extracts have a sort of proven track record for thousands of years, without the very obvious sword of Damocles hanging over their use. On the other hand, recent news media reports alleged that among the side effects of newer drugs, against Malaria, were possible suicidal tendencies.

On the other hand maybe, just maybe public awareness of our nutritional and general intake predicament is slowly but surely increasing as illustrated in a national daily publication's recent cartoon. It depicted a lion and it's cub on top of a bluff surveying the savannah below for prey, when they spotted a couple of very obese tourists on safari wading through the brush. The Lion trying to coach the cub on the art of hunting, turns to the cub and says: "Never eat one of those beasts. They're full of Transfats, banned substances, and toxic chemicals",

Everything breathed

As far as everything breathed, your senses, your common sense, and if need be your instincts/feelings as well, (unless you choose to overrule them) can easily let you know what may be avoided and what encouraged.

Speaking of inhaling choices, some smokers in Europe, in order to counter the health warnings on cigarette packs, apply stickers or (pack) sleeves encouraging smoking. It is no surprise that over the past ten years Americans smoked less while Europeans smoked more. Recent medical reports indicate that second hand smoke causes cancer in our pets as well. Respiratory diseases are multiplying, geometrically and indiscriminately, affecting infants to the very aged, with some form of asthma leading the parade. Breathing polluted air, as repeatedly reported by medical science, can be dilapidating and eventually deadly, but this is also a matter of choice. Some may not be surprised that a recent study revealed that air pollution can also cause heart disease, and this was apparently more obvious among commuters crawling daily on super-crowded freeways, streets and roads

Being on the lookout for "signals" and letting your "Philharmonic" guide you, may very well prove, once again, that it just won't fail you.

Physical activity

Yet another recent medical "eureka" is that exercising shrinks the risk of depression (among many other things). Healthy Mind in a Healthy Body, again.

Proceedings of the National Academy of Sciences reported that a study on adults between ages 58 to 78 indicated that exercising showed increased brain activity and decision making capacity while performing several tasks, improved by eleven percent.

Most are aware that "the use it or lose it phenomenon" fully applies to our muscles, joints, and other organs and parts of our bodies. Basically, it is activity versus inactivity. More recently, studies by Dr. Benjamin D. Levine, director of the Institute for Exercise and Environmental Medicine at Presbyterian Hospital in Dallas, dramatically reconfirmed that "the use it or lose it phenomenon" is at least equally true if not more so for the heart as it is for leg muscles and joints. Physical activity will maintain a vigorously functioning heart, healthy and young independent of chronological age, as well as contribute to maintaining youthful attributes in general for much longer. The alternative is, apparently, faster and premature ageing, and of course, heart attacks and their consequences. Indications are that exercising, at any time and at any age, can potentially reverse the ravages of a sedentary lifestyle. Dr. Levine may not have stumbled into Ponce's fountain of youth, but rather made his point that exercising is one heck of youth elixir and, particularly, for the heart. Who knows, it might even cut down on facelifts.

A study conducted at the Massachusetts General Hospital and Harvard Medical School have determined that people with osteoarthritis in their lower joints improved their condition markedly more through the physical activities of "functional training" i.e. holistic, than those engaged in just muscle-strength training. Physical therapists and operators of functional training centres around the country also found that it is as well beneficial to those suffering from rheumatoid arthritis, Parkinson's, cardiovascular problems, and several other ailments. The benefits are even more valid as one gets older. It is amazing but sad that many are convinced that as they grow older they will inevitably lose flexibility, strength, muscle mass, balance, and co-ordination at the very least, talking about needless but destructive preconception and prejudice. It might sound like a Murphy's Law for the elderly. However some may realise that it is nothing more than the ubiquitous law of "Use It Or Lose It" applicable to all and may be more so as one gets older. Because over time through evolutionary lifestyle changes and probably preconceived notions, physical activity practices and habits get altered and mainly curtailed and whatever is not used is lost and rust seeps in. Many have often heard that "older people get clumsy and fall and break all kinds of bones etc." The "legendary" justification being that with age their balance and co-ordination went down the tubes and osteoporosis made their bones brittle. One may wonder if the outcome would be different if they had kept utilising all their functions to the fullest. Maybe balance and co-ordination would have been there and muscle mass would have protected the bones. All bones are inherently brittle, the protection by the muscles often makes a difference just like the Styrofoam in a cyclist's helmet

The body *always* signals in multiple and varied ways that it welcomes physical activity. As far as everything pertaining to physical activity, it may be quite similar to the previously mentioned "single diet." Just do whatever YOU (not anybody else) love to do and enjoying doing it. Here too, loving and enjoying is the binder that keeps everything "together," not unlike the way gravity keeps the Universe "together."

Some folks love to run, and others hate running unless they are chasing a ball, etc. There are those for whom jogging, instead of being fun becomes almost cultish a struggle and a strain, with misery, agony, and stress, written all over their faces while jogging. However, they persevere mostly out of fear that if they don't, they will endanger their health and life according to what they have been told and yet they might even call this perseverance "Will Power," i.e., choosing to do something they do not enjoy. That may sound like an oxymoron, and embracing the oxymoron as usual, leads to self-contradiction and internal conflict and finally stress.

That, or a similar kind of "Will Power," might remind some of a 4WD SUV straddling a super snow bank and all four wheels spinning all out with the driver sitting there while persistently (with disciplined "will power") flooring the gas pedal, until eventually the transmission, the differentials, and/or the engine collapse. Others attempt, i.e., compel themselves to feel good after a run as a result of deciding to believe that they successfully "disciplined" themselves to jog for the "cause." It brings to mind that old Irish Catholic joke: *"If it's fun, it must be sinful, if it's a pain in the butt, it must be holy."*

Some on the other hand may be of the opinion, though, that THE ONLY THING "SINFUL," IS NOT ENGAGING IN WHATEVER IS LOVING, JOYFUL, AND FUN, and this is definitely no joke.

> To some of those who viewed the popular scientific documentary movie "What The Bleep Do We Know"? it might seem that the movie does indeed demonstrate palpably the above, in addition to confirming the old "healthy (joyful?) mind in a healthy body". Nothing motivates, energizes, and empowers, as much as loving, enjoying, and having plain fun passionately. If there is something else, it would appear that it has not been thought of yet. Some may choose to get real, and replace the old *"No Pain No Gain"* with "No Joy No Gain." Maybe Confucius was not that confused after all when commenting about JOY.
>
> *It is everywhere and the know how is all that's needed to extract it*

Jack Welch former chairman and CEO of General Electric Co. wrote that the requirements of leadership consisted of four essential traits:

1   An overabundance of **E**nergy.

2   The ability to **E**nergize and motivate others.

3   Have the **E**dge and courage to make tough yes or no decisions.

4   The ability to **E**xecute, i.e., get the job done.

All engulfed by genuine passion.

Mr. Welch insists that the foundation of the above must consist of:

- Integrity.

- Intelligence with a strong emotional component and broad based maturity.

Some may wonder if the above was but a description of the late Great Communicator, Ronnie.

What Mr. Welch recommends, with authoritative experience for leading people and organizations, may seem to some that it is just as valid in leading one's life, while Being In Charge of one's self.

Some could possibly sum up Mr. Welch's recommendations as follows:

- Acknowledging your uniqueness, your absolute Free Will/Power of Choice of choice, and taking into consideration the law of Cause and Effect.

- Walking the talk a la Socrates.

- Energized motivation through passionate loving, enjoying, and having fun.

The "Little Corsican" said it well, *"twenty-five percent of the power of an army is its force of arms, and seventy-five percent of its power is its motivation."* Some automotive fans may compare motivation to the high-octane fuel that provides a "Mach 1" acceleration to a Corvette Z06.

Loving and enjoying is the precious applause for your "Philharmonic." The confirmation by one's feelings/ intuition may further provide the "encore" applause after applause.

To some, it would seem that Ronald Reagan was aware of the above. Many have dubbed him The Great Communicator, but maybe The Great Motivator would have been more appropriate. Maybe being such a powerhouse of motivation, he was able to communicate and motivate America when it needed it most.

When he took office the country was deeply traumatized by Watergate and Vietnam, and people were practically spitting at our uniformed men and women. Besides a depressed economy, high unemployment, inflation, and interest rates, that were in orbit, President Carter talked about the pain of the "malaise" factor. American workers were being told, by the pessimists and the self-flagellation fans, that they were way inferior to their European and Asian counterparts, in productivity, efficiency and quality.

A clinical diagnosis might have indicated that we were wallowing in an ocean of inferiority complex and possibly heading for the depths of depression.

The Great Motivator made us whole again. He restored our morale, self-confidence, self-esteem, optimism, and patriotism. Americans travelling the world, once again started flashing, with pride, their US passports. This miracle of American Renaissance was maybe far more vital than the dismantling of the "Evil Empire," or the boosting of the economy and even national defence. No other president seems to have accomplished such a Mission Impossible. Motivating is indeed supreme leadership.

State of mind

Some may consider that an open mind is shackle free and provides peace of mind. An open mind may function more efficiently and harmoniously as the "conductor of the Philharmonic." Basically, an open mind is a mind that is adaptable and can face anything and everything without the shackles of preconception and prejudgement, which are but self-imposed limitations that may eventually lead to stress.

Epictetus, the first century AD Greek stoic philosopher aptly stated, *"Men are tormented with the opinions they have of things, not by the things themselves."*

Healthy Mind In A Healthy Body again, the Women's Health Initiative, which was the largest study of postmenopausal women (over 93,000 participants), clearly showed that depressed women had a fifty-percent risk of developing heart disease and/or dying from it. This study confirmed other similar studies around the world. Another study showed that men who lose their temper are more prone to heart trouble. Plato epitomized it well: *"He who is of a calm and happy nature will hardly feel the pressure of age, but to him who is of an opposite disposition youth and age are equally a burden."*

Lifestyle

Some may find that a healthy lifestyle starts with being in charge of one's self, thus bypassing self-contradictions and the resulting internal conflict, which leads to stress at the very least. Being in charge of one's self, allows one to be in charge of one's health as well.

And, when one's "Philharmonic" is swinging away making "joyful music" one may be at peace with one's self and, therefore, automatically choose a lifestyle free of excess, devoid of stress, and full of the loving and joyful, which may truly jive with the way our founding fathers put it "the pursuit of happiness."

11 - AGEING, PARADOX OR SUPERSTITION?

Just days prior to the 2004 presidential elections, it was announced that Chief Justice Rehnquist of the Supreme Court was being treated for thyroid cancer. Predictably, the news media immediately seized this information and kept regurgitating it while trying to politicise it by injecting it into the election campaign through speculation on various consequences. Eventually they regurgitated on the medical aspect of Mr. Rehnquist's cancer by interviewing several experts in the medical field. The consensus revolved mainly around the fact that the current Supreme Court members' average age was the oldest ever in its history. Also mentioned was the fact that three other justices had also suffered from cancer, etc., etc.

However the common thread that kept being repeated was that these four cancer cases were to be expected "as people beyond 60-65, the more they age the more likely to get cancer and other diseases". This intimation seemed to support the widely spread popular notion that the longer life's chronometer ticks away the sicker and more dilapidated one must get while drowning in a (although) well intentioned ocean of chronic medication and hypochondria

As previously mentioned, this fearsome myth/notion could seem to some as tantamount to being sentenced to be buried alive and tortured till the last breath and last buck.

Paradoxically, at the same time there is no dispute from any quarter, that the Big Bang's most "magnificent wonder", the human being a.k.a UBB's most magnificent creation, the-bio chemical, electro-mechanical contraption that is a:

- self-sustaining,

- self-regenerating

- self-repairing,

- self-healing,

- self-computing

- "Gizmo of Ultimate Perfection", GUP for short.

Probably most AARP members may be "Trekkies" or at least familiar with the original Star Trek series and some may even appreciate the typically Vulcan, Mr. Spock. He might reason that if we are inherently into automatic self-regeneration, and self-healing, etc., then the mere ticking of our life's chronometer should be (at least ideally) irrelevant to our "state of repair or rather disrepair"... UNLESS the process is somehow disrupted and or impeded, in one word "**overwhelmed**".

As Dr. Andrew Weil seems to indicate this **overwhelming,** causes most if not all of our health problems and since the GUP is also self-computing (read as our inherent absolute Free Will/Power of Choice) we are the authors of almost all of the **overwhelming**, most of the time, of our mind-body complex.

If one were to ask Mr. Spock "but why the aged?", he might respond with "they have been busy longer at **overwhelming** their mind-body complex". Remember the saying "Drop by drop, a drop of water may eventually pierce granite"

Tragically, all this ill health that is "expectedly" hitting the aged, seems now to also afflict in some degree the young as well, and increasingly so. How do you explain this, Mr. Spock? Without even raising his eyebrows, Mr. Spock might respond by quoting Sherlock for starters "Elementary, my dear Watson... the newer generation(s) have started the **overwhelming** much sooner than the older generation(s). For some maybe even before emerging from the womb. Also this **overwhelming** now seems to be even more excessive as compared to that of preceding generation(s)".

This **overwhelming** may be perpetuated mainly via the following:

o Everything ingested

o Physical activity or lack thereof

o Lifestyle

o Excess

o Stress

All of which as previously illustrated are subject to one's Free Will/Power of Choice.

To some it might seem that there are mainly Two Options.

Option one, (seemingly by far the most prevalent) is to capitulate to the superstition about ageing and lay down and wallow in that dreadful swamp of sickness, suffering, dilapidation, despair and depression, while choking on chronic medication and treatments. All the while hoping against hope for the mythical silver bullet, and mumbling resignedly "it comes with the territory" or "*c'est la vie*" while simultaneously contemplating buying cheaper drugs in Canada.

Option two is to cease and desist from **overwhelming** one's body and mind and instead, start reversing any "**overwhelming**". Just as Dr. Andrew Weil has stated on Larry King

"*You want to facilitate healing, not prevent it*".

To succeed, it is essential to listen to your body. As Bill Clinton confessed, he learned the hard way after his quadruple bypass surgery, (and now he seems unequivocally committed to always really "feel his body's pain" ASAP..), then establish full communications between mind, body and feelings/ instincts and lastly fine tune "Your Philharmonic".

Some may find that it all comes down to plain common sense. Senior citizens due to their seniority and long experience should be the least likely to deny it and thus discrediting Cartesian philosophy. René Descartes, the seventeenth century French philosopher-mathematician who came up with "*I think, therefore I am*" said the following about common sense:

"Common sense is the most widely shared commodity in the world, for every man is convinced that he is well supplied with it".

Finally, Mr. Spock in bidding his adieux, might conclude by paraphrasing Bill Clinton: "It's the overwhelming stupid!" followed by his ubiquitous Vulcan "V" hand sign and the salutation,

"Live long and prosper"

However there are possibly those who may doubt the validity of Mr Spock's logic and maybe even welcome a debate. Unfortunately the Planet Vulcan is more than a couple of blocks away and space travel cost still quite prohibitive.

For a possible validation of Mr Spock's position they might consider the Chancellor Emeritus at Baylor College of Medicine in Houston Texas, Dr Michael De Bakey. Dr DeBakey is a fit as a fiddle 96 year *young,* Always *superactive,* working long hours as energized as ever by his love and dedication to the Hippocratic Art. Maybe Duracell in an effort to increase the sales of longer lasting batteries, should fire the Energizer Bunny and make Dr DeBakey their poster boy.

Dr DeBakey is renowned for his research, inventiveness and pioneering in cardiovascular medicine. According to the Journal Of the American Medical Association (JAMA) "many consider Dr DeBakey to be the greatest surgeon ever". He hung up his scalpels at a youthful age of 91, presumably because they became worn and dulled and also to devote more time to research and teaching.

He is still not on any medication whatsoever and at today's gas prices he is probably saving a bundle not having to drive across the border to Canada to fill prescriptions. When it comes to Aristotle's Golden Moderation Rule he is a big time fan and would probably endorse the aforementioned **Option two.**

Some may picture those who choose Option One as disintegrating jalopies held together by unravelling threads, while they may picture those who choose Option Two as valuable, precious vintage classic and above all functioning automobiles. While it would seem that Dr DeBakey is one vintage class act, let us remember GOD's/UBB's original specs, although each unique, we are all created equal with Free/Will Power of Choice and unlimited possibilities.

However, some (of all ages) who may be "allergic" to good old plain common sense, perhaps they could ponder over Harry Truman's cautioning about common sense: "You either have it or you don't, and if you don't you might as well not get out of bed in the morning."

12 - HEALTH ARCHITECT IN CHARGE

If you so choose, a healthy mind in a healthy body may be achieved effortlessly and automatically, since your "Philharmonic" may outperform any mainframe on the planet including IBM's newest ASCI Purple, which will be operating at one hundred teraflops or trillions of floating-point operations a second, making it the fastest on the planet.

On the other hand, IBM's ASCI may eventually become a necessary "hardwired" crutch for anyone who chooses to disband the "Philharmonic," and instead surrender unconditionally to the myriad recommendations (quite often contradictory) along with the resulting stress and endless symptom swapping, with outcomes as tragic as those reported daily in the media.

All this may become irrelevant, should you choose to be the architect in charge of the health of your body and mind and build on the inherent six key factors affecting your physical and mental health. As the architect in charge, you may at any time if **you** so choose, "subcontract" with the subcontractor(s) of your choice, i.e., all sorts of health "givers," from physicians, to therapists, to pharmacists, or what appears to be Dr. Weil's holistic favourite, Integrated Medicine.

Being in charge of your health could, however, produce a fattening side effect; it may fatten your wallet. Among many other expenses, some may no longer choose to keep investing in the latest gadgetry that supposedly will safeguard one's health.

One of the latest gadgets is allegedly a hi-tech toilet that automatically analyses urine and then it e-mails the pertinent findings to one's physician. Maybe the next related invention would be a hi-tech toilet tissue that once used, it can be faxed to the friendly neighbourhood proctologist in exchange for a faxed back invitation (no RSVP necessary) to the next colonoscopy gala.

Yoko Ono and John Lennon, during their seven-day, bed-in peace protest in 1969 in a hotel in Montreal, produced the hit *"Give Peace a Chance."* If John was still around today, and took one look at the pernicious state of our health, he might very well protest with an even longer bed-in and come out with an even bigger hit, "Give (Your) Health a Chance."

13 - KEEP IT SIMPLE STUPID

Be In Charge (Of Yourself and Your Health)*, It's Free Of Charge* is not about religion, theology, ideology, abstract spirituality, the supernatural, fads, or any kind of dogma, unless one chooses to make it so.

It does not prescribe, recommend, or promote products, diets, exercises, systems, procedures, and treatments, or any books dealing in "what to do, when, and how." Some of the Lemming Syndrome persuasion, though, might appreciate being told "what to do, when and how," as it provides the illusion of denying their Free Will/Power of Choice, the ultimate self-fooling.

Simply put, you do not have to do anything, only what you choose to, since choice has always been yours, is always yours, will always be yours, and never, never anybody else's.

It is simply about three simple, self-evident reminders of:

- Who we are.

- Our inherent Free Will/Power of Choice

- The health we were designed/created to enjoy.

Simplicity may very well be Divine Elegance, or for the Zeus Club members, Elegance of the Gods, most likely Olympian.

However, for those who may be unfamiliar with either God or Gods, they may just appreciate the *"Keep It Simple Stupid"* principle, which Henry David Thoreau must have been a fan of when he exclaimed, *"Simplify, Simplify."*

These self-evident reminders can be seconded by a kaleidoscope of publicly available common knowledge that is acceptable by many if not most. This knowledge and information may be anecdotal, factual or established. It could be ancient, historical or even current. With points of reference, be they findings, facts, news, plain common sense mostly devoid of intangibles and the abstract, lastly every day life experiences.

As Wise Soly, you know the wise guy who fooled around with the Queen of Sheba (and no, she was never employed as an intern in Soly's Temple), purportedly said, *"There is nothing new under the sun."* That may have possibly been translated much later, and directly, from ancient Hebrew/Aramaic by Yogi to *"Déjà vu all over again."* Maybe Mel Gibson could possibly verify the accuracy of the translation. These basic reminders consist of:

1. WHO YOU ARE is to "KNOW THYSELF" as suggested by the inscription at the Oracle of Delphi, and which may basically translate into:

   - *Each is unique.*

   - Each is equally endowed with the absolute Free Will/Power of Choice.

Through this simple reminder and the choices

(situations) presented to us incessantly, one may choose to grasp the ever present equal opportunity for an unlimited potential, that may only be limited by our self-imposed limitations. One may choose to function in health just as designed and created by the Big Bang itself, i.e., perfectly, and rendering irrelevant the myriad recommendations, dos and don'ts, while doing one's own thing in health, and lovingly, joyfully and with lots of fun.

2. *YOU ARE ALWAYS THE SOLE CHOOSER (CREATOR) OF YOUR EVERY THOUGHT, WORD AND DEED AND ALL SUBJECT TO THE UNIVERSAL LAW OF CAUSE AND EFFECT* (i.e., natural consequences).

By simply acknowledging that YOU are the author of ALL YOUR CHOICES, both those you choose with responsibility (i.e., taking into consideration effects/consequences), and those you choose without responsibility, you are therefore in charge of Yourself. Consequently self-contradictions/internal conflicts, fear, and stress, may become null and void.

3. FULL TIME, DIALOGUE AND INTERACT– ION BETWEEN YOUR MIND YOUR BODY AND YOUR INTUITION/FEELINGS.

By Simply fine tuning the "PHILHARMONIC" AND POURING OUT THE "MELODIES," free of cacophony and external static" one may find that the "Philharmonic" can be of great help in guiding your Free Will/Power of Choice towards one's greatest benefit.

The above three reminders may lead you unerringly to Be In Charge of Yourself and Your Health.

 IT IS AS SIMPLE AS THAT AND JUST AS EASY, while it is also totally FREE OF CHARGE AND EVEN FREE OF EFFORT.

There are some however, whose philosophy possibly somewhat masochistic, might be expressed as "why do it the easy (and simple) way, if you can do it the hard way. The underlying simplicity of the Big Bang appears to support those whose philosophy is the self-evident "why do it the hard way, if you can do it the easy way."

There are also some, as observed by many, who resist change and are even terrified by it and will doggedly cling to the status quo whatever that may be. The irony is that the whole Universe is all about ceaseless change and motion, or as Heracleitus put it, *"All is flux, nothing is stationary."* Some, therefore, who may have forgotten about who they are and about their inherent and absolute power of Choice/Free Will, may be afraid to remember as it might disturb their familiar "comfortable" status quo. They may want to revisit Plato's parable about a bunch of guys captive in a deep, dark, cave labyrinth. It might prove quite inspiring.

A rough approximation of Plato's parable is about some men held captive in a dark and deep labyrinth of caves and pathways. They were fascinated and terrified by the moving shadows that flames of a near by fire cast on the cave walls. They felt totally at the mercy of these moving shadows, and terrorized by the menacing monsters, which their thoughts or imagination conjured them to be. Finally, one broke loose and said, "Enough is enough. I'm getting outa here," and that was *his choice*. He invited the others to escape along with him. They refused, and that was *their choice*, saying his escape attempt was suicidal at best, and his fate would be worse than death. At least here, they felt relatively secure while they benefited from the familiar light and warmth of the fire.

Finally, after what seemed an endless trip of frustration and fear in the dark, strewn with all kinds of dangers, he perceived a pinpoint of light far ahead and above. He advanced toward the light and finally emerged from the cave into a bright, blue sky by a beautiful white, sandy beach and clear, turquoise waters and a green, pine forest nearby, etc., etc., but above all FREEDOM. Eventually, he mastered his feelings of joy about his liberty, and immediately thought of rescuing the others. He again risked life and limb to go back and lead them out. To his surprise, they would not believe his experience, they told him he must be hallucinating, and that they were quite content to remain secure and warm in a place they were familiar with. Evidently that was *their choice; their choice* to limit themselves.

Well over 2000 years later, Elbert Hubbard somehow summed up Plato's parable as follows:

"FREEDOM IS THE SUPREME GOOD. FREEDOM FROM SELF-IMPOSED LIMITATION."

Those who are In Charge of themselves and their health will likely agree with Elbert. They might also feel a greater appreciation and derive more joy from old Blue Eyes' hit, *"My Way,"* as well as Edith Piaf's hit *"Je ne regrette rien."* On the other hand, "Frère Jacques" (Chirac) though, might not enjoy the latter as much, following Saddam's dental check-up, compliments of Uncle Sam.

Some of those, who are being more and more in charge of themselves and their health, may feel inclined to exclaim what Julius Caesar uttered at the end of his Tour de France(unlike Lance's),*"VINI, VIDI, VINCI,"* Julius's "Vinci" was all about real estate acquisition and people subjugation. The interpretation of Vinci for those who may be "In Charge" could very well be:

Learned + Evolved + Contributed + Enjoyed = VINCI

According to the KISS principle, possibly, the lowest common denominator of the **Three Reminders** in just two words, is the inscription that greeted visitors at the ancient Oracle of Delphi:

"KNOW THYSELF"

Once reminded of who you are, and have taken to heart the Delphic suggestion, you may consequently through your power of choice, choose to Be In Charge Of Yourself. Then, and only then, you may also choose to Be In Charge of Your Health, following which, joy, fun, and the pursuit of happiness may become pure gravy. If the Delphic suggestion sounds "All Greek" to some of you, and still on the lookout for the proverbial silver bullet, seek no more, YOU ARE IT!

You may find that it is demonstrably based on self-evident common sense amplified by sequential logic, to which Aristotle might give a thumbs up. As for the non-members of the Zeus fan club, they may be reminded by the first chapter in Genesis, where UBB, (oops..,) GOD gave mankind dominion over everything on Earth. As per good old plain common sense it stands to reason that having dominion without Free Will / Power of Choice would be oxymoronic. Not even the 9th Circuit Court of Appeals in California declared GOD an oxymoron, just unconstitutional that's all.

In either case you may well choose:

THE JOY AND THE HEALTH OF BEING <u>IN CHARGE</u>